This is a beautifully written s
Kate's difficult cancer journe
sibility of meeting God in n
ration into meditation and spiritual gruw.....
all. This is a book not just for those facing traumatic times but
anyone who wants to seek a closer walk with God.

Jude Mackenzie, author and former communications
adviser at 10 Downing Street

A brave and ruthlessly honest account of a journey that took
Kate to death's door several times – and yet more profoundly in
touch with God than she had ever known. It's not an easy read
as we travel with her through mind-blowing pain and anguish,
but it is ultimately a life-enhancing and joyous tale of getting
to the very end of oneself. Kate finds God there in the depths
before, beneath and beside her, gently bringing her to a completely new way of praying, of being, and of connecting with
the one she has come to love more than life itself. I was deeply
moved and challenged.

Michele Guinness, writer, broadcaster and speaker

The apostle Paul writes that revelation comes through the Spirit
not the mind. It's in the ravaged depths of cancer that Kate ex-
plores these ideas, through experiences of the Spirit, the poetry
of Scripture and the wisdom of mystics and sages who have
gone before. Her reflections are beautifully crafted and sensi-
tively shared, taking us all on a journey into the shocking brokenness of humanity and the overwhelming embrace of God.

Revd Dr Tania Harris, author and director
of God Conversations

Kate Nicholas describes her experience of cancer with typical directness and honesty. But *To the Ocean Floor* is no misery memoir: always curious, Kate shares with her readers the profound spiritual journey that she travelled alongside her long walk through the valley of the shadow of death. Her account of the strength she drew from the Christian contemplative tradition is inspiring, uplifting and ultimately hopeful.

Sarah Meyrick, novelist and director of the Church Times Festival of Faith & Literature

In my opinion, *To the Ocean Floor* is Kate's most profound written work thus far. As Kate shares her journey of healing through cancer – again – the glory that permeates every facet of her journey is Jesus – his presence, his love, his grace. Kate shares her intimate pursuit of a divine connection with our loving God through deep contemplation and meditation on his divine Word. No matter how deep the darkness of our soul, Jesus is our light in the midst! He is our comforter, our helper, our peace. May the anointing upon this book stir within its readers' souls, and may they personally be filled with the knowledge of the glory of the Lord, as the waters cover the sea (Habakkuk 2:14).

Cindy Cox, teacher, author and leader of US-based healing ministry JesusChristHealsToday.com

Wow, what an incredible story! I have followed Kate's writing online, read her previous books and hosted her guest blogs on my website, but didn't realize how much suffering she faced in this most recent cancer journey. It was fascinating to read how she was drawn into powerful encounters with God when her body and mind spiralled into the 'watery depths'. I was very interested to learn how much meditation and mindfulness have helped her too. Kate is a great writer and has incredible yet humble insight that we could all do with reading and reflecting upon. I heartily recommend this book.

Claire Musters, author, speaker and
host of the Woman Alive Book Club

Kate Nicholas takes us with her as she spirals to the darkest edges, and finds God there. Beautifully written, compellingly honest, incredibly moving.

Emily Owen, author and speaker

A gripping account of Kate's latest experience with cancer – how and why does someone manage to contract three different types of this mutating disease? With powerful writing, she describes the indescribable: the numinous; the Creator; her loving God. Her poetic sharing of her experience on the ocean floor led me to wonder and awe. A memoir to ponder and consider; one to read while receiving from Kate's deep sharing of herself and her journey while joining her in praise to the unknowable God who makes himself known.

Amy Boucher Pye, spiritual director and
author of 7 Ways to Pray

To the Ocean Floor is an immersive journey into the depths of human experience through a second cancer diagnosis, with Kate as our experienced navigator. Learning to breathe in the depths of shock and trauma is a gift, and it's a treasure we find in this second part of Kate's story. On every page you will find candour, humour and beauty.

Ruth O'Reilly-Smith, broadcaster and author of God Speaks

Part cancer diary, part spiritual memoir, *To the Ocean Floor* is a powerful account of the richness to be found at the borders of life's journey. Kate Nicholas writes with an almost forensic precision so that both aspects of this book – the medical and the spiritual – sing with authenticity. It is rare enough to find such a powerful story of cancer and faith: rarer still to find it described in writing of such quality.

Gerard Kelly, author, speaker, poet and
co-founder of The Bless Network

Facing another round of cancer and complications, Kate weaves her personal story together with the teachings of Christian saints and mystics, ancient and modern, to show us how she learned to pray through hardship – and invites us to pray along. Reading *To the Ocean Floor* gives the embodied intimacy of listening to a friend tell you her story of survival, bearing witness to God's healing presence with her in prayer and Scripture.

This is Kate's best book so far. As her own faith grows deeper, she calls us to go with her to the depths – through fear, via prayer, to love.

Revd Jennifer Mills-Knutsen, senior minister
at American International Church in London

To the Ocean Floor

A second cancer journey
and a gateway to a profound
connection with God

Kate Nicholas

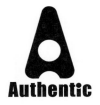

Authentic

First published 2023 by Authentic Media Limited,
PO Box 6326, Bletchley, Milton Keynes, MK1 9GG.
authenticmedia.co.uk

British Library Cataloguing in Publication Data
A catalogue record for this book is available from the British Library.
ISBN: 978-1-78893-300-1
978-1-78893-301-8 (e-book)

Cover design by Mercedes Pinera
Printed and bound by CPI Group (UK) Ltd, Croydon, CR0 4YY

In recognition of the wonderful staff of the UK's National Health Service (NHS) whose compassion, professionalism and resilience never fail to amaze me

Preface

This book is not a theological treatise on the nature of prayer but rather tells the story of how having cancer opened me up to a vivid inner experience of our transcendent, immanent Creator. It is also an account of my personal exploration of a contemplative tradition that dates back to the dawn of Christianity and seeks an intuitive connection with God. Before I began my cancer journey, I knew nothing of this tradition and I don't pretend to be expert on the subject, but I hope and pray that my story may inspire and encourage you to also be still and know that he is God (Psalm 46:10).

Contents

Preface   ix

Part One Embarkation   **1**

1 The Call   3
2 Waiting   9
3 Numinous   17
4 Bitter Pill   26
5 Rapha   30
6 Decisions   43
7 Carcinos   52
8 Hope   59
9 Doors   65

Part Two The Voyage   **79**

10 Setting Sail   81
11 Adrift   87
12 The Depths   95
13 Light   96
14 Silence   99
15 A Spacious Place   104
16 Holy Ground   110
17 Ancient Paths   120

18	Kingdom Glimpses	125
19	Limbo	136
20	Solitude	143
21	New Rhythm	151
22	Exploration	157
23	Shoreline	171

Part Three Arrival   **185**

24	Black Dog	187
25	Trust Fall	201
26	Anticipation	210
27	Travelling	218
28	Aftermath	227
29	Destination	234

Epilogue	239
Afterword	247
Resources	250
Bibliography	253
Contact the Author	256
Notes	257

You hurled me into the depths,
into the very heart of the seas,
and the currents swirled about me;
all your waves and breakers
swept over me . . .
The engulfing waters threatened me,
the deep surrounded me . . .

Jonah 2:3–5 NIV 2011

Deep calls to deep
in the roar of your waterfalls . . .

Psalm 42:7

The ocean floor is one of the last great unexplored wildernesses on this beautiful planet.

We know less about the deepest parts of the ocean than we do about the stars above. We have explored more of the surface of the moon than we have the great expanse that exists beneath the mystery of the waves, and we have more accurate maps of the surface of Venus and Mars than we do of the ocean floor of our own planet.

But if we could descend deep down into the mysterious depths, there we would find life – as, far from the rippling sun, existence takes on new forms, familiar only to the Creator. There light cannot penetrate but life persists.

Part One

Embarkation

1

The Call

I'm in another room when the phone rings, shattering the silence of the morning. I immediately recognize the number on the screen, and my heart skips a beat. An efficient disembodied voice explains briskly that I need to go back to the hospital for more tests after some 'suspect' findings on a routine mammogram. I feel the blood drain from my limbs, replaced by a profound sense of déjà vu.

The line goes dead, I place the phone on my bedside table, waver unsteadily and then fall heavily to my knees.

I can feel shock coursing like electricity through every atom of my body, numbness creeping from limb to mind – until only one thought persists: *I'd almost got used to the idea that I was going to live.*

The day before, I had marked my fifty-eighth birthday, a milestone I had once thought beyond my grasp. I'd spent the day wandering the local fields and woodlands, warmed by the first sun of early spring, wrapped in the comforting presence of my husband and children. Together we had celebrated another year of life gone by, twelve more months of precious memories made.

I no longer dread birthdays. In fact, my attitude towards the passing years has utterly transformed since my first cancer

diagnosis seven years ago. Whereas once I viewed each com-
memoration of my birth as a step closer towards mortality, these
days I view each birthday as a testament to the persistence of
life.

The 'cancer years' have changed me. My body is now
criss-crossed with the tell-tale tracks of surgery and my long
blonde hair is gone, replaced by a closely shorn grey crop.
When I was first diagnosed with cancer at the age of 51, a
friend of mine gave me a butterfly brooch that had belonged
to her late mother, and told me: 'I want you to have this because this period of your life will be hard but at the end you
will emerge like a butterfly out of a cocoon . . . You won't be
the same, but something different and beautiful.' I suppose I
could have grown my hair again and dyed it, but somehow the
boyish crew cut that emerged post-chemotherapy seemed to
testify to a transformation that runs very deep. Each morning,
as my shorn head rises from the pillow, I celebrate the day,
saying: 'This is the day that the LORD has made, and I will
rejoice and be glad in it' (see Psalm 118:24).

Then came the phone call.

Many of those who survive a cancer diagnosis have to learn
to live with a sword of Damocles poised over their heads; to
acclimatize to the creeping fear that the cancer, once banished into exile, will make its stealthy return and send us once
again to the brink. Survivors must remain vigilant, keeping
a weather eye out for any potential symptoms without suc-
cumbing to hypochondria.

My health has never been particularly robust but, until cancer came, there had been no discernible underlying disease;
rather, my ailments had tended to be of the common-or-garden
variety – broken bones, strains and twists, appendicitis,

migraine, irritable bowel syndrome (IBS), mild asthma and repeated chest infections. None were life-threatening, but these issues were numerous and visited me with monotonous regularity, undermining and frustrating my attempts to live life to the very fullest.

My father once reflected that 'my spirit was too big for my body'. In my relentless determination to get the most out of every day on earth, I tended to push myself beyond the ability of my body to cope. As a child I was rather frail and shy but was still determined to climb every tree, to ride my bike at full pelt and, on horseback, to gallop like the wind. My enthusiasm was never matched by ability, but I was undaunted and, after every fall, would pick myself up and get back in the saddle. As an adult, I continued to fling myself into new experiences in apparently reckless defiance of potential danger. It wasn't that I was fearless – in fact I could be quite timid in the face of real danger – but whether paragliding or solo backpacking in South-East Asia, I was determined to push beyond my comfort zone.

Whenever I was ill I was always determined to 'overcome' any physical limitation, tending to adopt a 'mind over matter' approach to my health. When viruses struck, I would struggle into work, unwisely spreading germs in my wake, and when pain reared its head I would attempt to walk it off. But in my early fifties the pain had become too intrusive to ignore and, when I was diagnosed with stage IV breast cancer, my local general practitioner (GP) told me wryly that I could have done with being more 'hypochondriac'.

Following my initial cancer diagnosis, I had tried to walk a fine line between hyper-vigilance and sensible precaution, and in the immediate aftermath of chemotherapy, surgery and radiotherapy I had religiously checked myself almost daily; but, as the days turned into weeks, then months and finally years, I had begun to relax. As the almost unbearable intensity of the experience began to give way to a more reflective existence, I had started to acclimatize to the extraordinary idea that against all odds I was going to live – until the fateful phone call.

Shaken, I remain crumpled on the bedroom floor, like a puppet whose strings have been cut, and try to rationalize away the portents. *Perhaps they just didn't get a good image and need to repeat the mammogram. Perhaps they have simply found some scarring. Perhaps . . .*

When I eventually rouse myself from my torpor I feel a desperate need to escape the confines of the house and to get out into the open air, so I head out into the morning sun in a bid to stride off the lurking terror – relying on action to overcome anxiety. I head up the lane that runs from my house through the ancient hedgerows and gently rolling landscape of north Buckinghamshire. The calm beauty of my surroundings feels incongruous, a reminder that life goes on while we contemplate our mortality.

It was this lane that first convinced my husband and me to buy a home in this village. Our house is not grand but affords wonderful access to the surrounding countryside, and for over twenty years now I've headed out in all weathers up the single-track lane that gently rises up above the house, carving a path between the wheat fields, drystone walls and blackberry bushes. The lane leads up to a Palladian alcove that sits high on the hill above the cluster of pale limestone cottages below; an architectural folly, built in 1753 by the lord of the manor for the local poet William Cowper, and known locally as Cowper's Alcove. Nestled among ancient chestnuts, its tiled roof and whitewashed pillars protect walkers from the elements, affording them a spectacular view over a patchwork of fields rolling down to the market town of Olney.

From this vantage point I have witnessed the yearly changing of the seasons: golden waves of wheat giving way to scarred post-harvest earth, and snow-covered ridges melting to reveal the first green shoots of returning life. Through the spring, summer, autumn and winter, I have come here to reflect, to try to make sense of life, to dream, to remember and to connect to something bigger than myself. It's a place that naturally seems to lend itself to prayer, providing a sense of separation and perspective as the morning mists rise above the distant roofs below.

Now I sit in the alcove frozen in shock, the dappled sunlight playing across the worn paving stones beneath my feet, phone in hand. I desperately want to ring my husband John, but I'm conscious that there's little he can do right now and I am reluctant to shatter his day. So, for now, I'm alone with the reality that the trajectory of our lives may once again be changing.

By the time my husband returns home, the sun has disappeared over the horizon. I share the news and watch the colour drain from his face. I immediately feel a terrible and irrational guilt at having introduced such uncertainty into his life again. Over the past few years, he has lived through not only his wife but also his mother and father being diagnosed with cancer, and I can see the toll this has taken on him. As the person at the centre of the storm, I had been caught up and relentlessly carried forward by the tide, while those around me were left feeling bereft and helpless, watching on the shoreline as I was battered by the waves.

That night John and I make the decision not to share our concerns with the children until we have a clearer idea of what the future may hold. Our eldest child is now a young woman with a master's degree under her belt, and a career that has taken her halfway up the country, while our youngest is experiencing all the potential and challenges of adolescence. When I was first diagnosed with cancer back in 2014, they were just 16 and 10 years old respectively; old enough to understand what was happening but far too young to deal with the emotional turmoil. At the time we had tried to protect them from the worst realities, but both have undoubtedly been scarred by the experience, and the thought of dragging them back once again into the darkness of doubt is appalling.

So, we wait.

2

Waiting

The Hebrew word used for 'wait' in much of the Old Testament is *qavah*, which means to actively wait with anticipation of what God will do. To *qavah*, we simply have to be patient and be willing to 'stay where we are and live the situation out to the full in the belief that something hidden there will manifest itself to us'.[1]

There certainly is a lot of waiting involved in a cancer journey. Waiting for interminable tests, results, treatments, meetings and phone calls, all of which carry the potential to radically alter your life and the future of those closest to you. Waiting is such a hard task when you have been told that there may be a time bomb ticking away within your cells. In the absence of information, one's mind tends to work overtime, filling the void with dark imaginings.

But a time of waiting is also a time of potential. We enter a liminal space where all things are possible because they lie beyond our control – and while we wait, we stand on holy ground.

The days until my appointment pass at a painfully slow pace. Time takes on an elastic quality when you are faced with a potential cancer diagnosis. When you're caught between the desire for knowledge and the need to postpone the moment of certainty, four days can seem like an eternity while also passing in the blink of an eye. I throw myself into work, trying to fill every moment before the appointed hour, knowing that gaps in activity provide too much time to speculate.

When Friday eventually arrives, I wake with the dawn and linger in the warmth of my bed for as long as possible, trying to hold on to the moment. While I remain under the covers, I am in limbo and can simultaneously imagine a reality in which life continues and another in which it's potentially cut short by cancer, but eventually I have to rise and face the day.

I make a cup of tea, and prise my protesting teenager out of her room, propelling her out the door and towards the school bus. Then, in the quiet, I open up my devotional. The scripture for the day is a familiar passage from the Old Testament book of Jeremiah:

> 'For I know the plans I have for you,' declares the LORD, 'plans to prosper you and not to harm you, plans to give you hope and a future. Then you will call upon me and come and pray to me, and I will listen to you. You will seek me and find me when you seek me with all your heart.'
>
> Jeremiah 29:11–13

These words were written as part of a letter that the prophet wrote at God's command to the exiled Israelites in Babylon, but the promise is timeless and today feels like a personal benediction – a message of potent promise and power – for which I am profoundly grateful.

Over the years I've been amazed by the way in which pieces of Scripture seem to find you when you need them most. It's as if God's word speaks directly into your situation, providing you with exactly the comfort, reassurance or guidance that you need at that time. In the Bible we are told that 'all Scripture is God-breathed' (2 Timothy 3:16). The words of the Bible were recorded by humans over many centuries and, as such, are coloured by their historical world view (which is why it is so important to understand the context in which they were written), but they were inspired by God and contain universal and eternal truths which continue to speak into our lives.

It is often in our darkest moments that we are most alert to the fact that God's word is still 'living and active. Sharper than any double-edged sword, it penetrates even to dividing soul and spirit . . . it judges the thoughts and attitudes of the heart' (Hebrews 4:12). I know that the Bible is God's way of speaking to us, so I decide I will keep this promise with me, buried deep in my heart in the days ahead. I then go downstairs to find John and show him the passage and, while he does not necessarily share the depth of my belief, his surprised smile seems genuine and I know that he is not just humouring me.

I met my beloved husband back when I was 29 years old, still wore size 12 clothes, had a luxurious mane of blonde hair and was living in a backpackers' hostel in the leafy Sydney suburb of Glebe. He was an Australian hippie who had been cycling solo around the continent for the past eighteen months. In Sydney for one night only, to get his bike fixed, he was celebrating his birthday with a group of newly acquired friends in the fashionable waterfront Rocks enclave close to the Harbour Bridge – and I was invited. It was love at first sight. We were not, however, an obvious match; I was a successful public relations executive on a break from reality, while he was seven years younger than me, had longer hair than mine and no discernible source of income. Yet there was an immediate, profound and undeniable connection, and the next day he didn't leave Sydney as planned.

In the early days of our relationship we occasionally discussed the subject of faith. We established that I was a seeker on a globetrotting spiritual quest, still trying to work out my relationship with God, while he told me that he'd been brought up in the Roman Catholic Church, the child of Lithuanian refugees, but no longer attended mass. Yet, despite the differences in our spiritual outlook, it quickly became clear that we shared deeply held values about prioritizing experience over money, and relationships over material success, and that in a fundamental way we looked out at the world from the same place.

Over the years, however, as my own faith deepened, it had begun to pain me that my husband wasn't sharing this experience. At my request he had come along to some services at our local Anglican church, but I could sense that he never felt comfortable. Nevertheless, despite the changes that my growing faith has wrought in my life, he has remained ever by my side and supported me as I explored my vocation.

Over the last couple of decades I have tried to evangelize my husband in various ways but have come to realize how presumptuous it is to assume he doesn't have a relationship with God, just because his relationship isn't the same as mine. I now recognize that it's sheer arrogance to presume that his eternal salvation relies on my actions. But it means so much to me this morning as together we bow our heads and pray.

Once we arrive at the hospital, events move with speed. I'm asked to change into a revealing hospital gown and am steered towards a dimly lit waiting room. As the UK is still in the grip of the Covid-19 pandemic, John is told to wait with the other partners outside. It's a necessary precaution but one which only serves to reinforce the fact that this can be a lonely journey.

Initially I am alone in the waiting room, but one by one other women appear, clutching their fears tightly. Most are middle-aged, but there's one young woman who must be no more than 20 years old. All of us have been called back for further investigations and the anxiety in the air is palpable. I am drawn into a conversation with a woman next to me who asks me if this is my first time. At first, I'm not sure if I should reveal that this is a road I have travelled before (it's hard enough to deal with the initial diagnosis, let alone the prospect that the cancer might return one day), but then I realize that the sheer fact that I am here to tell the tale is, in itself, a testimony of hope. As we talk, something in my manner seems to reassure her.

When it's my turn, a chirpy young mammographer fixes a copy of my latest mammogram onto a wall-mounted digital screen, the negative revealing in stark contrast two areas of suspect tissue. The suspicious areas are only small, which explains why they had escaped my regular checks, but I can see the shadows quite clearly. Still, I cling on to the hope that these are not tumours, but my reluctant brain cannot help registering the fact that the suspect cells are not in the previously affected left side but in the right. If this is cancer, it has commuted.

Throughout the process, the mammographer adopts a forced tone of jollity while I say silent prayers and hold on tightly to a small wooden clutch cross. This small olive-wood cross has been with me since the very beginning of my first cancer journey, and I've clung on to it through countless scans, X-rays, consultations and even surgeries. By now it must have absorbed considerable amounts of radiation and I'm surprised it doesn't glow green in the dark, but in the midst of the storm it has felt like an anchor for my soul, my knuckles turning white as I press into the dark-grained wood.

When we are finished, I am guided down a corridor of doors, and as I turn the corner I spot a familiar face. In one of the doorways stands the consultant radiologist who walked me through my very first investigations seven years ago and first confirmed my suspicion that I had cancer. During the very first scan, she had informed me that there was a large mass of cancer and that it had spread. While I had appreciated being told the full facts, it was a hard pill to swallow. However, a couple of weeks later, when she performed my 'benchmarking' scan, she had seemed very puzzled. As she ran the scanner over me for a second time, she asked whether I had already started my chemotherapy. At the time, I had thought it a rather odd question, given that this was my pre-treatment scan; however, it was only as I left that I turned to enquire why she had asked that question. To which she responded, 'Well, it's just that it doesn't look as bad as the first time I saw it!' All I could say was, 'There's a lot of people praying for me' – and from that conversation, hope and a friendship was born.

Now here she is again, waiting and smiling as I make my way down the corridor.

'How great to see you!' I enthuse without thinking.

She grins broadly, lifts her arms as if to hug me, but thinks better of it. 'You too!'

The nurse accompanying me looks rather bewildered as we chat away, caught up in the moment, but gradually the incongruity and the gravity of the situation sinks in and the tenor of the conversation becomes more muted.

The radiologist sits down at her computer and, pointing to the image on the computer screen, explains: 'These two areas weren't there when you last had a mammogram eighteen months ago. As you have had cancer before, we are going to have to take this seriously.' She tells me that I need to have two biopsies and the insertion of small metal clips at the sites of the potential tumours.

I've had a difficult relationship with needles since the age of 18 when a group of medical students massacred my right hand in a botched attempt to insert a cannula. As a child I had always associated vaccinations and blood tests with the sweet reward handed out by our local GP, but after this incident I developed something akin to needle phobia, and the next time I was approached by a needle I passed out, much to my subsequent embarrassment. Thankfully, I no longer actually faint at the sight of needles but, as the nurse prepares to inject my breast with a large syringe of local anaesthetic, I feel distinctly nauseous.

During the procedure I feel no pain but am conscious of tissue being taken from the tumours and feel like an apple that has been cored. Then, during the insertion of the metal tags, I have the distinct impression I am being stapled. But the business is over and done with relatively quickly and, armed with a cup of tea, I regain a modicum of equilibrium. Then we talk.

My radiologist friend leans forward, looks me directly in the eye and says, 'I know from the book you wrote about your previous cancer journey that one of the things you appreciate about me is that I give it to you straight . . .'

Time stands still. Gazing around the room, I take in the apparatus of prognosis, and the doom-laden image on the screen, and her words seem to pass through the air in slow motion: 'I'm sorry, but I have to tell you I am pretty convinced that this is a recurrence of the cancer.'

When the meeting is over, I wander in a daze out into the hospital, lost in thought and a labyrinth of corridors, until I finally emerge into the damp spring morning and the arms of my husband. We sit in the car park, rain running down the window screen. Until this point, he has tried to convince himself that the problem was a mere administrative error but, as I share the events and conversations of the morning, my 6-foot 6-inch bear of a husband dissolves into tears like a child. All I can do is hold him, tell him how much I love him, and reassure him that I will do anything I can to be with him and the children for as long as possible.

Once again, however, we make the decision not to worry the children until we have had a final confirmation that this is indeed cancer. Perhaps it's cowardice, this pushing the telling down the road, but they have already been through so much. So, for now, at least, they have no idea of the storm that is forming over the horizon.

That night when I finally drift into unconsciousness, I dream that I am on a raft cresting the gentle swell of the Ionian Sea heading towards Corfu – a place that for me represents both freedom and death. This is the island that my aunt Theresa fled to in the 1950s, setting up home with her artist lover Christo, and where I laid her to rest after she succumbed to the ravages of cancer. This is the land that I now sail to in my sleep.

3

Numinous

I haven't always been a Christian, and my faith journey has been far from simple. When I was very young, I seemed to have an instinctive understanding that there was more to the world than meets the eye. A solitary child, I would spend hours roaming the countryside alone, content with the sense that I was being watched over and accompanied by some undefined but benign presence.

I was brought up as a Baptist by my mother, but was very influenced by my father – an intense and eccentric poet who could be described as an anguished agnostic. Today he might be diagnosed as bipolar, but in those days he was left to his own devices, trying to make sense of himself and the world. He had an extraordinary mind which ranged far and wide in his search for meaning. He was obsessed with the work of the Swiss psychoanalyst Carl Jung who had a complex relationship with God, and his own relationship was equally complicated. My father had a good understanding of the Bible, and could readily quote from it, but he was also fascinated by the spirituality of the East and would pore over the ancient Chinese divination text the *I Ching* as well as *The Tibetan Book of the Dead*.

I was only 11 years old when he told me that life was no longer worth living, and I spent most of my teenage years terrified that he would commit suicide. With each of his descents into darkness I found it increasingly impossible to reconcile my father's pain with the idea of an omnipotent loving God.

The church teaches that God is both transcendent and immanent – that he exists beyond and independently of the known universe and is beyond our understanding or perception, but also that he exists within the universe, pervading all of creation, and is perceivable and knowable. According to the Bible, he is all around us and within us, and knows everything we do and our every thought (Psalm 139:2–5), but to me God seemed very distant and lacking in empathy – an absent landlord. I wrestled with the question of why such an all-powerful, all-loving God would allow my father to suffer so much, but I failed to find an answer in the church. So, in my late teenage years, I turned my back in anger, and walked away.

Filled with righteous adolescent outrage, I started to attack anyone who professed belief – including my mother, whom I regarded as gullible, naive and deluded. The relentless positivity of Christians irritated me like a hair shirt and seemed to fly in the face of rationality. I wanted to hold up the woes of the world to them like a mirror that would reveal their credulity, and began to seek out evidence of the worst aspects of humanity to make my argument. I joined the campaigns against nuclear armament and vivisection, and would point to the threat of nuclear annihilation and the suffering of animals as proof that God was not in his heaven and all was not right with the world.[1]

At the age of 18 I left home to study for a degree in Fine Art at the University College of Wales in Aberystwyth, a seaside town in west Wales with a distinctly New Age vibe. The town and the surrounding countryside were full of colourful characters, many of whom subscribed to an eclectic range of beliefs. I met Wiccans and wanna-be Druids, Buddhists and Taoists, as well as some who were attracted to the beliefs of the early Celtic Christians. As an art student I was rather intrigued by the Celtic belief that God can be experienced through appreciation of his creation. The idea that we could connect with this thing called God without even stepping inside a church rather appealed to me and, as I walked the heather- and sheep-covered hillsides and shell-covered shoreline, sketchbook in hand, I was reminded of that sense of the numinous that I had experienced in early childhood before my militant rationality took over.

After completing a master's degree, I moved to London and went to work for an advertising agency promoting everything from kettle-jugs to car seats. My twenties were something of a spiritual wasteland, but by the age of 29 I had become utterly disillusioned with the rampant consumerism that I was paid to promote. I felt trapped in a life that wasn't mine but didn't have the courage to get out – until, one day, I had an epiphany. As my mind wandered in an interminable meeting about a forthcoming consumer goods promotion, a thought penetrated my consciousness with the force of a bullet: 'I don't know what God wants me to do with my life, but this isn't it.' It was a thought that was impossible to ignore, so I handed in my notice, sold just about everything I owned and bought a round-the-world ticket.

I left in search of a more meaningful future, and my journey turned into something of a spiritual quest. The all-pervading spirituality of the Indian subcontinent came as a shock after the rampant secularism of my homeland where religious belief is increasingly seen as a fringe preoccupation of the eccentric few. Fascinated, I began to explore the religious roots of this remarkable land. I made my way north to the ashrams of Rishikesh and up to Dharamsala, the Himalayan home of the deposed Dalai Lama, where I sat among the scarlet-robed monks listening to gurus of the Mahayana tradition. Further south, I wandered the glittering temples of Thailand, trying to find out more about Theravada Buddhism. I was entranced, seduced by a world view so alien to my own, but ultimately I realized that I was merely a tourist and that my spiritual home lay elsewhere.

I travelled on to Australia, where I met John, and together we returned to the UK where I entered the secular world of the newsroom and spirituality took a back seat to my career. I revelled in the world of journalism and rapidly climbed the ladder, becoming editor and ultimately editor-in-chief of a magazine called *PRWeek*. I regularly covered the machinations of Whitehall and the spin emanating from Downing Street, and became a regular TV commentator on current affairs and news programmes. I was a professional cynic, and the more voracious my criticism, the more the magazines flew off the shelves. But after a while disillusionment crept in, and once again I was plagued by the thought that there must be more to my existence than this: *If there is a God, then this cannot be what he intends for my life.*

It was a series of chance conversations that instigated my exploration of Christianity. Over a period of a few weeks, I had a number of encounters with Christians who spoke in pragmatic terms about the grounds for their faith. Intelligent and widely read, they challenged my preconceptions and my curiosity was piqued. Everything I'd known to date about Christianity seemed to fly in the face of rationality, but I began to realize that I needed to take a more informed view. So,

I bought myself a New Living Translation copy of the Bible and started to read it during my commute to work. Over the following year I read the sixty-six books of the Bible cover to cover – twice – while huddled into a crowded train carriage. I was horrified by some of the atrocities recorded in the Old Testament but mesmerized by the person of Jesus, who challenged me to the core. If Jesus was indeed God-incarnate, then this was a very different deity from the one I had rejected in my youth for his lack of empathy.

I also turned to some of the great intellects to find out how they were able to reconcile what they knew of the world with their faith and, after exploring various theologians, came to the same conclusion as C.S. Lewis – that Jesus' claims preclude the option of regarding him as simply a great moral teacher, but force us to decide whether he was either insane, a liar, or telling the truth, no matter how difficult that option may be to swallow. I realized that the man I had met in those ancient pages spoke with greater sanity about humankind, the world and its ways than any other thinker in history, and his unwillingness to lie – even to save his own skin – led him to the most terrible of deaths. So, the only option left to me was to accept the extraordinary, unavoidable and world-shaking truth – that this man was God.

I have always been an action-oriented individual so, once I had accepted that truth, I knew I had to do something about it – to put my faith into action. I started to attend my local Anglican Church of St Peter and St Paul, a beautiful thirteenth-century edifice where John Newton, the former slave trader turned clergyman, once preached and wrote the haunting anthem 'Amazing Grace'. At first the formality of the services felt alien, but I soon found the rituals comforting and grounding. I therefore gave myself up to the liturgy and, as I did so, was filled with a profound sense of awe.

I came to treasure my time in church but soon realized that I couldn't be just a Sunday Christian and that I needed to commit my life more fully. So, in my early forties, after the birth of my youngest child, I gave up my lucrative and respected job in the media to join the Christian aid agency World Vision. Suddenly I was surrounded by Christians of multiple denominations, and prayer and worship became part of not only my personal but also my professional life.

Responsible for global communications across the 100 countries we operated in, I travelled to some of the toughest places in the world, where I encountered the most extraordinary faith-filled individuals. I met people who had virtually nothing and no semblance of control over their destiny but who, in the face of grinding poverty and the most terrible natural disasters, maintained a deep sense of trust that God had a plan and a purpose for their lives. Everywhere I went – from the flooded slums of Jakarta to the remote rural villages of Malawi, from the container camps of north Mexico to the HIV clinics of the Dominican Republic – I could see Christ at work, wandering through the fetid alleyways, bending beside the broken backs of workers in the barren fields and comforting those for whom hope was all but lost.

Then in my early fifties came the pain in my shoulder – easily explained away by a recent sharp encounter with a car door – and the racing heart which I dismissed as a symptom of stress and my globetrotting, jetlagged lifestyle. But by the time I finally heeded the subtle warnings, the cancer had moved in, set up home and was busy building extensions. The cancer had spread beyond the original site and into my lymph system up under my collarbone, to the mediastinal area around my lungs and into the pericardial sac around my heart, and as such was inoperable.

The prognosis was not good but, as I absorbed this information, I found to my amazement that I was not afraid. I was desperately sad at the thought that I might have to leave my family, and I was daunted by the potential pain of the death process, but I was also inexplicably calm.

It was the psychotherapist Jung, with whom my father was so obsessed, who proposed the idea that human beings could be understood as different psychological types. His ideas were developed by Catherine Cook Briggs and her daughter Isabel Briggs Myers into an assessment tool for determining personality types that is known as the Myers-Briggs Type Indicator (MBTI) and is widely used around the world. According to Myers-Briggs, we all naturally sit on a spectrum somewhere between the opposites of introversion and extroversion, sensing and intuition, thinking and feeling, judging and perceiving. According to the assessment, my personality type is an ENTJ, which stands for extroverted, intuiting, thinking, judger. This personality type gets their energy from engaging with the wider world. They also have an intuitive streak, but are very rational, prizing conclusions of the head rather than the heart, and tend to be very action-oriented with a need to take control of situations.

Some tendencies sit further along the spectrum than others. For example, my extroversion is one of the more obvious aspects of my personality as I am undoubtedly energized by interacting with the outside world, while my 'intuitive' streak is less obvious, even to myself, and tends to be overpowered by my 'thinking' tendency. Certainly, my approach to the challenges of life has always seemed to be driven by my head rather than my heart and I have always demonstrated a 'judger's' need to be in control of every aspect of my life, including my health. In fact, for years, I had taken every measure possible to stave off the crisis that I now faced. I had barely drunk any alcohol. I didn't smoke and lived mainly off superfoods such as kale and quinoa while avoiding processed foods and red meat. I juiced on a daily basis and powerwalked my way around the local lanes – but apparently it had been to no avail. I had still succumbed to cancer.

I had worked so hard over the years to secure the future of our little family but was finally in a situation completely out of my control. It was as if God was saying to me: 'Stop holding on so hard, and just let go.' I could almost feel him prising my fingers off the tiller and when, exhausted, I finally loosened my grip, God was able to do something extraordinary. But now, after six years of exile, it seems that the cancer may have returned and all I can do is wait, watch and pray.

The minutes, hours and days pass so slowly and I wait in anticipation for a sign that my plight has been noticed on high; but, after the first gift of the Scripture passage from Jeremiah, the celestial radio remains silent. Instead, I focus my attention on the family, but every interaction with my children takes on an almost unbearable intensity, heightened by their obliviousness to the approaching storm.

Then, twenty-four hours before my results appointment, I receive a random call from a representative of a secular association that represents small businesses; he wants to encourage me to take up membership. My first instinct is to politely nip the conversation in the bud, but then the cold caller seems to go off script: 'I really wanted to talk to you because we have two things in common – cancer and Christianity.'

The caller shares that his cancer, a rare sarcoma growing in the muscle and soft tissue of the leg, was found during a routine scan and that when the tumour, which was the size of a lemon, was excised, he lost so much blood that he ended up in intensive care, and subsequently had to learn to walk again. Curious, I ask him what this experience has meant for his faith. He thinks for a moment and then replies, 'Perhaps the Lord hasn't finished with me yet.' Adding: 'I'm convinced you will come through this. Like me, God has more work for you to do.'

The wait is almost over.

4

Bitter Pill

I already know what the surgeon is going to say before she opens her mouth. It's as if some primitive part of me has been preparing itself for what lies ahead but, until the words were spoken, I was able to hold on to the fantasy that cancer was a thing of the past, a memory buried deep, never to be resurrected. Now the words hang in the air in the space between us.

There is no easy way to be told that you have cancer. No sugar-coating that will take away the bitterness of the pill. 'It's cancer' are the words that no one wants to hear about themselves or their loved ones. John's tension is palpable. I can almost taste it on the air. My breath seems to pause and my pulse to slow, as time once again elongates. A multitude of questions jostle for attention: *Why now? How far has it spread? What does all this mean?*

At the beginning of the year, I'd been admitted to hospital with severe stomach pain and abnormal liver enzyme levels, the cause of which remained unidentified. At the time I was just relieved that the pain had subsided, but now the memory comes back to haunt me as I begin to make silent connections. *Has the original cancer come back and spread not only to the other breast but also to other parts of my body?*

The surgeon continues: 'It is grade three, and at present the lymph nodes look negative, although we are going to have to do another CT and a bone scan just to check that it is no-where else.'

When I was first diagnosed with advanced cancer in 2014, my oncologist had issued a dire prognosis and, when I unex-pectedly went into remission, the consensus of medical opin-ion was that my recovery, while remarkable, was simply a stay of execution. As I celebrated my healing, my oncologist had sought to temper my joyful optimism with dour warnings that it was 'only a case of *when*, not *if*, my cancer would return', adding that, as and when the cancer popped its head above the parapet again, it was most likely to make an appearance in my lungs, liver, brain or bones. For this reason, I had always dreaded the appearance of 'secondaries' elsewhere in my body.

Now I hang on the surgeon's every word. I know that the lymphatic system functions rather like the body's metro system and is capable of transporting cancer cells around the body, so I hold on to the hope that the cancer is still contained. But then she adds, 'It's actually a different cancer from last time.'

The cogs of my brain whirr furiously. 'What do you mean – a "different" cancer?!'

'Well, the last time you had cancer it was oestrogen recep-tor positive, but the two biopsies have come up as receptor negative.'

My mind works overtime trying to decipher what this means. My greatest fear has been spread of the original cancer, so now I wonder if I am being thrown a lifeline: *If the cancer is different, then surely it can't be a recurrence of the previous cancer and is less likely to have spread?* I've absolutely no idea whether there is medical validity to these assumptions but, as the rhythm of time resumes, I find that I'm able to be rela-tively pragmatic as we begin to discuss the next steps, which are going to be surgery followed by radiotherapy. Mercifully, chemotherapy isn't mentioned as an option.

Chemotherapy is a strange beast: tame for some, and for others aggressive in the extreme. I've known patients who have worked throughout their treatment, and others who have been brought to their knees, and even defeated, by chemo. When previously diagnosed with cancer my options were initially limited to chemotherapy as the tumours were deemed inoperable, so I'd embraced what I hoped would be a life-extending, if not saving, treatment. However, within a few days of commencing treatment on a drug called docetaxel, I was admitted to hospital with sepsis, and had drifted in a twilight world of semi-consciousness until my merciful recovery. Unwilling to risk losing his patient unnecessarily prematurely, my oncologist had then reduced the dose to a level which I found easier to manage.

The side effects of the treatment, however, took a heavy toll on me. The irony of chemotherapy is that it gives life by bringing death: scourging the cancer from our bodies by killing off healthy fast-growing cells, including red and white blood cells and platelets, as well as those that control hair growth – leading to the distinctive baldness of the cancer patient. It also attacks the cells that make up the mucus membranes of the mouth, throat and digestive system; as a result, even the air you breathe and the water you drink tastes as if it has risen up from sulphuric depths. In addition, the intense fatigue that chemotherapy can induce gives the impression that it is robbing you of your youth while it goes about the business of restoring life. It's a necessary evil, but not one that I relished the idea of experiencing again in a hurry. In comparison, surgery seemed like an easier option – even if, as suggested, I might require chemotherapy further down the line as a measure to prevent recurrence. This was a reality that I could face later on.

We go on to discuss the potential different types of surgery and I become baffled by the myriad of choices: lumpectomy or mastectomy, single or double mastectomy, mastectomy with implants, mastectomy with natural tissue reconstruction. I review the grisly menu like a diner struggling to make a choice of entrée, and eventually ask: 'What do you recommend?' I desperately want to be guided, to surrender the responsibility for myself to the expert sitting in front of me in this cramped office. I need an answer before I go back out into the world again and before I face my children.

The surgeon mentions the word 'lumpectomy' but then recommends that I have a single mastectomy combined with an implant reconstruction. I agree immediately. The surgeon seems somewhat surprised at how quickly I reach this conclusion, asking: 'Perhaps you would like to take some time to go away and think about this?'

But I grasp at what seems like a clear road map for my journey – I will have a mastectomy with an immediate reconstruction. The surgery will take place soon after Easter, which comes early this year, followed by radiotherapy. The plan seems sensible, the timeline manageable and the situation containable. It's a sensible and reassuring narrative that I can take back to my offspring.

I breathe a sigh of relief, and feel warmth flooding back into my heart. I think I'm beginning to see the detail of God's plan to give me a hope and a future. But, as I glance down at my left hand in which I tightly clutch my wooden cross, I notice that my palm is imprinted white with the pressure.

5

Rapha

During this period of waiting, the potential return of the cancer has been a closely kept secret between my husband and me. While the world has carried on around us, we have been existing in a cocoon of anxious uncertainty. But now that the words have been spoken and the cancer diagnosis has been confirmed, we need to share this reality with those closest to us, starting with our children.

When this storm last broke over our little family, the sense of calm that God instilled in me seemed to help my husband and children to cope, even as I faced potentially leaving them. And the fact that he delivered me, against all odds, from death no doubt sowed seeds of confidence that were now bearing fruit. However, I wasn't underestimating the impact that the news was going to have on my loved ones.

In the end, the conversations turn out to be easier than expected. As my eldest now lives at the other end of the country, we connect with her using FaceTime, which is not ideal. Not surprisingly, her initial reaction is one of utter shock. Visibly shaken, she says that she has to go away and compose herself but, by the time she calls back, her tone is pragmatic as she asks about the diagnosis and treatment plan. My 16-year-old is also very emotional when we first share the news, but my confidence seems to reassure her. I point out that it doesn't look as though I will need chemotherapy and that the treatment will all be over in a few months' time. But I can't hide the fact that our lives are going to be turned upside down again for a while.

As a family we had so many plans. Having been locked down for so long because of Covid, we were yearning for the restrictions to lift so that we could travel again. During our enforced isolation we had spent hours poring over maps, reading travel guides and dreaming about distant lands. I was particularly keen for us all to travel to Japan and was planning a research trip for my next book which would take me around the United Kingdom and as far afield as West Africa.

For most of my life I've travelled. I am, at heart, an explorer who revels in touring God's earth and witnessing the great diversity of his creation. Driven by a deep wanderlust, my husband and I have continued to seek out new places and fresh experiences and, paradoxically, when in motion I seem to be able to find a stillness and calm which too often eludes me in daily life. Perhaps it's the distance from the distractions of the everyday, the necessity of paring down your existence until it fits into a backpack, that seems to enable me to see God more clearly.

Now, the journeys we have dreamt of are not to be. However, while I may not be embarking on a physical journey, I recognize that what lies ahead of me is still in its own way a venture into the unknown. It certainly isn't an adventure I would have volunteered for, but for the foreseeable future I will, like all true explorers, be sailing uncharted waters.

I still feel a kinship with the ancient Celtic Christians, many of whom exhibited a God-driven wanderlust. (Perhaps the sense of connection emanates from my Welsh and Irish heritage. Certainly, whenever my father was exasperated by me, he would throw the accusation at me that I was 'such a Celt'.) These early Christians regarded all of life as a journey, a voyage into the great unknown in search of the mysterious rationale for our existence. For some, that journey was physical; St Patrick, for example, first landed on Ireland's shores as a slave but, after escaping back to Wales, he later returned to the land of his captivity as a missionary and is credited with converting parts of Ireland to Christianity. Other Celtic saints such as Brendan and Columba travelled in the opposite direction, obeying an Abrahamic-style command to leave their homeland, setting sail across forbidding seas in a bid to spread their particularly Irish brand of Christianity. But the journey that was most important to the early Celtic Christians was an inner one: a transformative journey of the soul – a quest in search of the Christ that 'dwells in us' and a true understanding of the self that dwells 'in Christ'. This too is a perilous journey, and I believe that this is the voyage I am now embarking on.

Before I set sail, however, there are preparations to be made. When I last embarked on the journey of cancer, I had taken a characteristically proactive approach. Despite the dire prognosis, I had decided not to give up hope and initially set about finding out all that I could about the disease and potential treatments. Early on, I went online and found a report in a respected medical journal which said that 85 per cent of people whose cancer had spread as mine had died within twelve months. After that I kept away from Google and realized that I had to be very careful about my reading material. I put aside the medical journals and decided instead to study in depth what the Bible had to say about healing.

In the early days, I was thrilled when I found the following verses in the Old Testament book of Proverbs:

> My son [or daughter], pay attention to what I say;
> turn your ear to my words.
> Do not let them out of your sight,
> keep them within your heart;
> *for they are life to those who find them*
> *and health to one's whole body.*
>
> Proverbs 4:20–22 NIV 2011, my italics

And as I immersed myself in Scripture, I found that one of the Old Testament names for God is Jehovah Rapha, which is variously translated as 'the God who *heals*, *repairs* and even *cures*'. This word is used sixty-seven times in the Old Testament, and one of the first times that God speaks to humankind he describes himself as 'the God who heals you' (see Exodus 15:26).

I also found out that the Greek word for 'to save' is *sozo*, which is used 110 times in the New Testament. Taken from an Aramaic term which means both to 'make alive' and to 'make healthy', *sozo* is a word that is vast in meaning, encompassing both spiritual and physical healing as well as complete wholeness and well-being.

In the prophecies of Isaiah, I came across a wonderful passage about the death of Christ, written about seven hundred years before he was even born:

> Surely he took up our infirmities
> and carried our sorrows,
> yet we considered him stricken by God,
> smitten by him, and afflicted.

But he was pierced for our transgressions,
    he was crushed for our iniquities;
the punishment that brought us peace was upon him,
    and by his wounds we are healed.

Isaiah 53:4–5, my italics

It's a passage much beloved by those facing medical challenges but, in the course of my study, I found out that it's only when you look into the original Hebrew of the Old Testament that you uncover the full richness and depth of meaning of this scripture. In fact, the Hebrew word for 'infirmities' is *choli* which also encompasses malady, sickness and disease. The word for 'sorrows' is *makob*, which means not only mental suffering but also physical pain. The term used for 'peace' is that marvellous Hebrew greeting *shalom* – which indicates complete well-being and wholeness of spirit, soul and body – and the word for 'healed' used here is *rapha*, one of the names of God. I realized with wonder that if you take the original Hebrew meaning, this scripture makes the incredible claim that Jesus, on the cross, carried not only our sinful natures but also our physical and mental suffering, paving the way for us to be made whole.

In the New Testament, I also pored over the thirty-one accounts of Jesus' healing of individuals, plus at least twenty references to mass healing in the gospels. As I read, I began to comprehend that the reason why Christ healed was to give humankind a glimpse of God's kingdom, a tangible sign of God's will on earth. That it was because Jesus *was* the Creator incarnate that he had this ability to control the elements – calming a storm and walking on water, multiplying matter in order to feed thousands, and transforming matter to heal diseases or even overcome death. With his coming, however, this power to transform wasn't limited to Christ. In fact, Jesus granted this power to transform physical matter liberally to his followers, initially sending out his inner circle of twelve disciples while giving them 'power and authority to drive out all demons and to cure diseases' (Luke 9:1) and then a further seventy-two of his followers armed with the ability to heal the sick.

Some believe that after Jesus' death such miracles of healing ceased, but the book of Acts records how the apostles Peter and Paul demonstrated the power to heal and even to restore life in the name of Jesus, 'the name that is above every name' (Philippians 2:9). The name itself wasn't magic; rather, it was belief in the authority, power, sheer goodness and compassion of the person of Jesus himself which transformed those who spoke it.

The letters written by Paul also speak of healing as one of the gifts of the Spirit that were manifest in the early church. The late John Wimber, a renowned preacher and healer who investigated the history of healing in the church, found that during the first four centuries following Jesus' death, manifestations of healing were common in the early church, which partly explains the rapid growth of Christianity at this time. Then with the establishment of the Orthodox Church a whole raft of saints were identified to whom miracles could be attributed – including St Peregrine (1260–1345), the patron saint of cancer.

Peregrine Laziosi's qualification for canonization rested on two miracles: the miraculous supply of wine and grain to the people in Forli during a time of severe food shortages, and his spontaneous healing from cancer. One of the Friar Servants of

St Mary in Italy, Laziosi was a man of deep holiness and strict discipline who vowed that he would only sit when absolutely necessary and remained standing even when he developed a cancer in his right leg. But his condition deteriorated to the extent where his physician told him there was no option but to amputate his leg. The night before the operation, Laziosi had a vision in which Christ touched his leg and, the following morning, when the physician arrived to perform the surgery, he could find no evidence of cancer. Laziosi lived on for another twenty-five years. When he finally died of a fever at the age of 85, hundreds of mourners, including those seeking healing, attended his funeral. Many healings took place that day and, in 1726, he was canonized by Pope Benedict XIII and is still considered the patron saint of all those suffering from cancer.

As the Middle Ages progressed, reports of such healings began to die off; but, from the Reformation to the twenty-first century, accounts of similar miracles have been steadily increasing in number, facilitated partly by the increasing ease of communication.[1] In fact, in 2018 the BBC published a survey which found that 62 per cent of adults in the UK believe that some form of miracle is possible today, and half of those questioned by the market research firm ComRes admitted that they had prayed for a miracle at some time.[2]

Contemporary miracles may not command headlines in the way that the parting of the Red Sea, the plagues of Egypt or the raising of Lazarus did, but my own experience and that of others I have listened to over the years convinces me that miracles – large and small – do still take place, and that, as we continue to unpick the mysteries of the universe we live in, we may in time better understand how God works through his creation.

Which is why I decided, back in 2014, that I would also pray for miraculous healing. I was particularly encouraged by Jesus' assertion in the Gospel of Matthew that 'if two of you on earth agree about anything they ask for, it will be done for them by my Father in heaven' (18:19 NIV 2011) and by his further assurance: 'If anyone says to this mountain, "Go, throw yourself into the sea," and does not doubt in their heart but believes that what they say will happen, it will be done for them' (Mark 11:23 NIV 2011). With rather simplistic fervour, I decided that I was going to cast this mountain of cancer into the sea and was determined to use every tool at my disposal to do so.

Every morning I would mentally strap on the full armour of God (as described in Ephesians chapter 6) so that I could take a stand against cancer. I would buckle the belt of truth around my waist, remembering that he is Jehovah Rapha, the God who heals, and would put in place the breastplate of righteousness, won through Christ's sacrifice, and remembering Isaiah's prophecy: 'by his wounds we are healed' (Isaiah 53:5). With my feet 'fitted with the readiness that comes from the gospel of peace' (Ephesians 6:15), I mentally took up the shield of faith and put on the helmet of salvation, praying for protection against fear. Finally, I took up the sword of the spirit, which is God's word.

At the beginning of this first cancer journey I had also come across a book, *God's Creative Power® for Healing*, by the American preacher Charles Capps, who writes about the power of speaking God's word into our life today. One of the terms used for 'word' in the Bible is *dabar*, which also means 'deed', thus indicating that God's words are creative. According to the creation account in Genesis, 'In the beginning . . . the earth was formless and empty . . . And God said, "Let there be light," and there was light' (Genesis 1:1–3). Capps claims that God's word continues to be creative today, that as we speak God's creative word it becomes part of us, and that: 'When you speak God's Word from your heart, then faith gives substance to the promises of God.'[3] The Bible tells us that 'the tongue has the power of life and death' (Proverbs 18:21) and God himself says that as his word goes out of his mouth:

> it will not return to me empty,
> but will accomplish what I desire
> and achieve the purpose for which I sent it.
>
> Isaiah 55:11

So, every morning, I would read healing scriptures out loud and, as I spoke God's word, my faith was strengthened.

I also decided to seek out a healing prayer group. This was not an easy move for me. As a former journalist, I was still very sceptical about some of the more charismatic elements of the church and, having spent some time working in the United States, had become very cynical about prosperity gospel preachers and healers who regularly appeared on television presiding over apparent miracles. The sight of audience members leaping out of wheelchairs and throwing away crutches while TV pastors asked for large donations had only fuelled my scepticism. I knew that instantaneous healings had happened in the past and even believed that they could happen today, but I also knew that few healings were this dramatic and sometimes took time to manifest. However, I reasoned that I had little to lose, so decided to seek out a reputable organization.

I made contact with a local healing prayer group through the London-based Christian Healing Mission and began to meet with the members regularly, particularly before treatments or scans. They would lay their hands on me, anoint me and pray over me, and the results took me by surprise. In fact, it's hard to express how powerful the experience was; at times it felt as if electricity was passing through my body and, one occasion, I had the distinct impression that the cancer was leaving my body and passing into the air like dust motes.

On one occasion, one of the healers asked me if I would like to engage in Encounter Prayer; this is a form of prayer developed by the Christian Healing Mission, who describe the practice as 'creating a space to meet with the living God for relationship, healing and transformation'.[4] Although I didn't have great expectations, I was curious, so I decided to give it a go.

The prayer leader began by praying to '*Abba*, Father' and then, as I closed my eyes, asked me where Jesus was for me at that moment. I have always found it very hard to visualize; whenever I've engaged in the kind of relaxation exercises where you are invited to imagine yourself on a beach or by a waterfall, all I ever saw was the inside of my eyelids. But within seconds a face appeared vividly in my mind's eye. However, it wasn't a face that I recognized. The person I saw in front of me was rather plain with dark skin, a large nose, coarse dark hair and a stubbly beard. It was not an overly attractive visage and far from the European image of Christ with his ethereal beauty, pale skin and long flowing locks that I had grown up with – but I knew that it was him. After a while, the face began to move towards me until we were nose to nose and then, much to my alarm, this ruddy countenance moved even further forward until it seemed to merge into my own. This personage had somehow become part of me.

Months later, in a doctor's surgery, I happened to pick up a copy of *National Geographic* which contained a feature about a facial reconstruction artist who had modelled the face of Christ based on available anthropological information. As I turned the page, I nearly dropped the magazine. Staring out at me was the face that I had seen in my rather unnerving encounter with Christ, down to the last detail. God knew only too well my journalistic need to see evidence and had used the very medium that I had previously worked with to counter my scepticism.

When, against all odds, I survived, I consciously committed my life to the Lord in gratitude. At the time, I wasn't sure exactly what this looked like, but I knew that I wanted to live every moment of every day dedicated to him. However, over the six years of glorious remission that followed, my initial fervour and my dedication to spending time in Scripture and prayer was gradually eroded as my days once again became filled with a relentless round of activity (even the experience of cancer didn't seem to have slowed me down).

More recently, my spiritual life has also suffered due to the closure of places of worship to prevent the spread of Covid. As an extrovert, being part of a church family and interacting with other members of the congregation has been an incredibly important part of my life. Christianity is an inherently communal faith; as difficult as it can be to fully comprehend, God has always existed not as a solitary individual but as three persons in a divine relationship. He *is* a community made up of the Father, Jesus the Son, and the Holy Spirit, and he is not only loving – he *is* love. The action of loving requires an object, which is why God not only exists as relationship himself but also made humans to live in connection with him and others. This is the reason the earliest Christian communities referred to themselves as the 'body' of Christ. God celebrates our individuality and our diversity, but we are also called to come together as his *ekklesia* or congregation, united in love. As the apostle Paul says: 'The body is a unit, though it is made up of many parts; and though all its parts are many, they form one body. So it is with Christ' (1 Corinthians 12:12).

For the past twelve months, however, as I write, church doors have been barred and for the first time in centuries we have been unable to gather, and I miss the act of communal worship and fellowship that so energized my faith. I yearn for my church family and feel like an ember that has been out of the fire too long. During lockdown, I've sofa-surfed various online church services, singing along to the worship songs enthusiastically and tonelessly, but it hasn't been enough. I realize how important the rhythm of church life has been to maintaining and fanning the flames of my faith.

So, in the absence of this community, I turn again to the example of the early Celtic Christians who were distinguished by their spiritual discipline and rigorous dedication to structured spiritual exercises – a 'rule of life' they referred to as 'green martyrdom'. The Latin root of the word 'rule' means a trellis, and the early Celtic Christians saw spiritual discipline as a trellis which provided a framework to guide and support their development throughout their lives. Now, looking to their example and the journey ahead, I realize that I also need some kind of spiritual discipline to keep me on track.

So, in preparation for the road, I decide to draw up a set of resolutions regarding spiritual disciplines: my own personal 'rule of life' as I go through treatment for cancer a second time. First of all, I commit to continue starting my day with Scripture, working my way through *The Bible in One Year* with the aid of an app created by Alpha founder Nicky Gumbel and featuring the resonant tones of David Suchet. I reason that, no matter how challenging the road ahead, at least I can listen to the Bible while lying in bed.

I also resolve to pick up again the discipline of reading healing scriptures in the morning, but decide that this time I will go a stage further and will commit key scriptures to memory, keeping God's word close to my heart. I will begin the process by learning the poetry of the Psalms – allowing their eloquent expression of both pain and hope to permeate my being.

In addition, I will follow at least part of the pattern of Daily Offices of the Church of England, reciting the morning liturgy and the evening Compline prayers, and will complement this with some of the beautiful prayers from the Celtic daily tradition, including the exquisite 'St Patrick's Breastplate':

> I arise today
> through a mighty strength,
> the invocation of the Trinity,
> through belief in the Threeness,
> through confession of the Oneness
> of the Creator of creation . . .
> Christ with me,
> Christ before me,
> Christ behind me,
> Christ in me,
> Christ beneath me,
> Christ above me . . .

Finally, like a warrior, I will once again put on the armour of God as I face the 'battle' ahead.

6

Decisions

As an ENTJ personality type, I have spent my life seeking certainty. While Jungian 'perceivers' are more able to wait to see how a situation plays itself out, often leaving their options open until the last minute, 'judgers' such as me are profoundly uncomfortable with anything nebulous or unresolved and tend to always be in a hurry to reach a solution or conclusion. I have wryly observed the wisdom of this analysis over the years, and now, once again, I can see how this personality trait is playing itself out as I deal with this situation; when my surgeon offered what seemed to be a conclusive course of action, I had grasped at the reassuring certainty, rapidly closing the door on other possibilities.

One of the big changes that has taken place in medicine over the years has been the increasing choice offered to patients, who are encouraged to participate in decision-making; a development that can sometimes leave you trying to make impossible choices. Seven years ago, after grinding my way through months of chemotherapy, I was offered a wonderful but difficult choice. Despite initially being told that my cancer was inoperable, my surgeon was amazed at how well the chemotherapy had shrunk the cancer and decided that surgery might be possible after all, with the aim of removing, if not all, then some of it. So, he offered me the option of either a lumpectomy (with radiotherapy) or a single mastectomy. The decision was mine alone to make. While some women go on to rebuild their bodies, I was also told that reconstruction wasn't an option at the time, given the spread of the cancer – aesthetic considerations playing second fiddle to efforts to lengthen my time on earth.

Back then, as I deliberated, I stood in front of the bathroom mirror trying to imagine myself with just one breast and, as hard as I tried, I just couldn't make peace with the idea. I feel ashamed for even admitting this, as thousands of women make the brave decision to undergo mastectomies every year, but I really struggled with the idea of an asymmetrical existence, no matter how short my life might be. I made light of the situation to family and friends and joked that, given my 'ample bosom', if I had the mastectomy I'd spend the rest of my life walking round in circles; but, after much soul searching, I chose to retain the breast, and had only one part cut away and the remainder irradiated.

Now, once again, I stand before the mirror and struggle. I had agreed so rapidly to the surgeon's suggestion without truly thinking through the implications. What the surgeon had proposed was an implant reconstruction, one of the simplest methods of reconstruction that can usually be carried out at the same time as a mastectomy. In some ways this is an attractive option because when you wake up from the anaesthetic your body still appears symmetrical. But as I contemplate this prospect, I feel increasingly uncomfortable about having the implant inserted into my body. I know that many live very happily with implants, and I tell myself not to be irrational, but I cannot shake the doubts.

The surgeon had also made a comment relating to the very remote possibility of developing another cancer called breast-implant-associated anaplastic large cell lymphoma (BIA-ALCL) as a result of having an implant. It's an infinitesimally small risk and I would have to be very unlucky indeed to contract this, but it is enough to feed the seed of doubt in my mind which continues to grow as the days roll by.

Eventually, I come to the difficult conclusion that I don't want to have an image-saving implant reconstruction. But then I also begin to ponder over whether I also rushed at the idea of a mastectomy. Doubt begins to work its way through my system like a virus. All the certainty that I carried out of the surgeon's office begins to evaporate and I begin to ponder: *Do I actually need a mastectomy at all? The surgeon didn't offer a lumpectomy, but she also didn't say that I couldn't have one, did she?*

I find it impossible to sleep and in the middle of the night I start researching comparative life expectancy after lumpectomies versus mastectomies, drawing up a spidery flow chart of the psychological and medical ramifications. When the morning finally rolls round, I phone the breast-care nurse and ask her tentatively if another lumpectomy rather than a mastectomy might be an option. Within a matter of minutes, the surgeon calls back. I expected her to be exasperated but she patiently walks me through the options.

It seems that the two tumours that have been identified and classified as hormone negative are in roughly the same area in the lower part of the breast, and if this is the only cancer then a lumpectomy might actually be an option. But then she says, 'We've also found a third area of tissue in the upper breast that looks a bit suspicious.'

My mental antenna twitches.

'It's only small, which is why we didn't manage to get a biopsy, but I think we need to find out what this is before we make any decisions. I know you are having the CT and bone scan but let's also get you in for an MRI scan.'

The last of the comforting certainty that I had taken away from our last meeting evaporates. I realize that I am once again heading into the unknown with further scans ahead of me, all of which may reveal further challenges.

At all the critical junctures of my last cancer journey, I had turned to the healing prayer group. In those days, we gathered in a small room in the local church that doubled up as an office and, wedged between filing cabinets and a makeshift altar, they would pray over me and lay hands on my broken body. Every time they prayed, the atmosphere became so charged that this humble setting transformed into a holy place. Now, once again, I yearn for the companionship of these prayer warriors and the comfort of that Spirit-charged place, but as the country remains in lockdown our only contact can be online.

The evening before my first scan, we gather on Zoom to pray. At first, I am rather sceptical about how healing prayer will work over Wi-Fi, but am amazed as, one by one, these wonderful women pass on to me scriptures that had come to them ahead of our meeting, including the glorious sweeping comfort of Psalm 46:

> God is our refuge and strength,
>> an ever-present help in trouble.
> Therefore we will not fear, though the earth give way
>> and the mountains fall into the heart of the sea . . .

vv. 1–2

As they pray over me from their various locations, I feel stronger and can almost imagine myself armed for the battle ahead, clothed in the armour of God, my wooden cross in hand.

Over the next week, I clutch this cross through a plethora of different scans and try not to imagine how much radiation we are both absorbing. The first scan is a computerized tomography (CT) to check that the cancer has not spread to other areas of my body. After several years of check-ups, this is such a familiar routine to me, but the experience does not lose its poignancy. Over the past few years, I found that in-between scans I was able to push the possibility of recurrence to the back of my mind, but each time you open yourself up to such transparent scrutiny you become aware of the possibility that your nemesis will be found to have spread, stealthily, silently, unseen by the naked eye. Cancer can be a silent killer, gradually eroding life while you are blissfully unaware of its progress.

As I lay myself down and the scanner whirs into life, I hold on tightly to my cross and remember the scripture I was given at the beginning of this process: "'For I know the plans I have for you,' declares the LORD, 'plans to prosper you and not to harm you, plans to give you hope and a future'" (Jeremiah 29:11), and I silently pray a traditional Celtic Caim prayer of protection:

Circle me, Lord
Keep peace within, keep harm without

Circle me, Lord
Keep love within, keep hatred without

Circle me, Lord
Keep hope within, keep doubt without

Circle me, Lord
Keep peace within, keep evil out

Circle me, Lord
Keep protection near, and danger afar

Circle me, Lord
Keep light near, and darkness afar

Circle me, Lord
Keep joy within, keep fear out

Circle me, Lord
Keep light within, keep darkness out

May you stand in the circle with me
today and always.

Adding for good measure:

Circle me, Lord
Keep health within, keep cancer out.

The next day, at a different hospital, I'm injected with gamma radiation and submit to a full skeleton scan to assess whether there are any metastases in my bones. Lying in the scanner, I occupy myself by reflecting on the reassuring scripture from this morning's daily prayer which feels too topical to be coincidental:

The righteous person may have many troubles,
  but the LORD delivers him from them all;

he protects all his bones,
> not one of them will be broken.

Psalm 34:19–20 NIV 2011

Amen!

Finally, on a Sunday afternoon, I make my way through an eerily empty hospital to have a magnetic resonance imaging (MRI) scan. Few people relish the idea of being injected into a metal tube and surrounded by noises akin to a jackhammer tearing up a pavement, and I am no exception. As someone who is slightly claustrophobic (for years I would walk up flights of steps rather than take a lift), the idea of being immobilized and encased in this way is fairly disturbing. However, given the situation, there is no alternative but to grin and bear it.

I lie down, am injected with a dye, and then inserted into the tube upside down, my head clamped in a brace to prevent any movement. I'm offered music but, unless I opt for heavy metal, any songs I choose are unlikely to be heard over the sound of the jackhammer. So instead, I focus on the solidity of the cross in my right hand, and pray that the scans will come back clear.

The cross is such an unlikely symbol of salvation, representing as it does one of the most hideous and agonizing means of execution ever dreamt up by humanity. It often strikes non-Christians as strange that the central symbol of a faith based on love is an instrument of torture. Yet it has represented a beacon of hope for millions down the centuries. I've always loved the familiar image of the Celtic cross, which can be seen in graveyards all over the British Isles, particularly in Ireland and Scotland, as well as on everything from jewellery to album covers. I have fond memories of standing on the ancient Hebridean monastic isle of Iona gazing up at the Relig Odhrain silhouetted against a cold blue sky – the circle encompassing the cross of Christ. It's such an ancient symbol, which harks back to our pagan past, but it was co-opted by Christians to represent the eternal love of God and the hope of salvation.

For Celtic Christians the cross was seen to hold immense power and was a symbol of Christ's victory over evil. He is *Christus Victor*, who 'having disarmed the powers and authorities . . . made a public spectacle of them, triumphing over them by the cross' (Colossians 2:15). In the tradition of the ancient hero sagas, Christ was seen by the Celts as the ultimate conquering warrior or *Dryhten*, and the cross is imagined as the scene of the ultimate battle. As such, the image of the cross itself was seen as having power over evil and was often invoked in prayer as a weapon to be used in spiritual warfare and for protection.

The jury is still out on exactly what causes cancer. Our genetic make-up, lifestyle and environment undoubtedly play a role but, when I asked the oncologist (a leading expert in his field) who treated my previous cancer, he said: 'Honestly, ninety per cent of the time it seems to be sheer bad luck.' I don't believe in luck or that cancer is the work of the devil, but I've seen enough cruelty in the world to be convinced that evil does exist and can invade our thoughts, undermining our relationship with God, who is good, and replacing faith with fear. So, as I lie in my magnetic field buffeted by pulsing radio frequencies, I pray the ancient Celtic prayer, 'Be the cross of Christ between me and all ill',[1] for 'the message of the cross is foolishness to those who are perishing, but to us who are being saved it is the power of God' (1 Corinthians 1:18).

Then, surrounded by the banging, whirring, clicking and beeping of medical science, I have the distinct feeling that Jesus is lying there with me in the scanner, body on body, soul on soul, without and within, speaking into my fear and telling me: *This isn't going to be easy but I am here.*

7

Carcinos

Cancer is one of the great levellers in life; no wealth, privilege or private healthcare policy can protect you from its ravages. Nearly all of us know someone who is currently being treated for, has recovered from, or has sadly died as a result of this malignancy. It is also not a new phenomenon, although we have undoubtedly contributed to its prevalence through poor diets, lifestyles and lack of stewardship of our environment.

The first documented case dates back to ancient Egypt, a papyrus from 1500 BC recording eight cases of tumours occurring in the breast (which makes breast cancer not only the most common cancer in the twenty-first century but also the most enduring). An Egyptian physician recorded that the cancer was not curable, but provided palliative treatment in the form of cauterization using a hot instrument called 'the fire drill'. But it wasn't until about a thousand years later that the ancient Greek physician Hippocrates named the condition, using the Greek words *carcinos* and *carcinoma* to describe tumours.[1]

These days cancer seems to be an omnipresent threat. At the time of writing, residents of four out of the eight houses in the cul-de-sac in which I live have cancer – a poignant illustration of the fact that around 50 per cent of us will be visited at some time or another by this condition. Even so, it's still always terrible to have to watch your nearest and dearest being ravaged by their errant cells. Over the years, I've seen far too many of my friends and neighbours diagnosed with cancer, the most recent being the husband of my closest school friend, Cheryl.

I first met Martin forty years ago when he began 'dating' my friend. He was 39 and she only 18, and the general consensus of opinion was that, given the age difference, the relationship was doomed to failure. Four decades later, however, the two of them were still together, having given life to three children.

In the early days of their marriage, I had the impression that Martin regarded me as a bad influence. In our twenties, while Cheryl was making house and bringing up children, I was living the high life in London, going out to a different club or gig every night after finishing work for the day in the ad agency, and whenever I went to visit their substantial Surrey abode, decked out in goth gear bought on Camden Market, Martin would watch me warily like a snake keeping an eye on a predatory mongoose. But as the years rolled by, the suspicion turned to mutual respect and eventually deep affection.

I came to love Martin dearly; he was undeniably a character and given to outrageous pronouncements and teasing humour that could easily be misunderstood, but I recognized in him the qualities that I so adored in my father: an uncompromising honesty, great kindness and determination to live life on his own terms. When cancer came calling, he adopted a strategy of stubborn denial and, apart from close family, few knew of his illness. When he confided in me that he had a tumour in his lung, my initial thought was that the cancer didn't stand a chance. At first, he seemed to weather chemotherapy with alacrity, cheerily cycling around the local town with his

Golden Labrador on a lead, heartily tucking into food and enjoying a couple of glasses of whisky every evening. But a year and a half on, Martin was undoubtedly fading. His appetite was diminished and he had now resorted to exercising the dog by driving round the local park in his Land Rover with the frustrated canine chasing the car.

Knowing that I had previously been through cancer treatment, he would occasionally call at odd hours to ask my advice: 'Why does everything taste so b****y awful? You lived on a diet of carrots, didn't you? I'm not doing that.'

As the prospect of cancer loomed over the horizon for me again, his wife decided to keep my investigations under wraps. He had been so distressed when I was previously diagnosed with cancer, and neither of us wanted to do anything to undermine his bloody-minded resilience. However, he and I kept talking on the phone until, one day, the conversation took a different turn.

Having discussed the frustrations and practicalities of hair loss, fatigue and chemo-induced constipation, Martin asks me: 'You believe in God, don't you?'

'Yes, I do.'

'And that has helped you?'

'It certainly has. It has given me amazing peace – even when I thought I wouldn't make it.'

'You weren't afraid?'

'I was so sad, and I really didn't want to leave John and the kids, and certainly didn't want to die, or be in pain. Sometimes that kept me awake at nights but, when it came down to it, no, I wasn't afraid.'

'Why not?'

'I think because I just *knew* really deep down that it wouldn't be the end, that there's more to come.'

I then tell him the story of my mother's last hours. My mother Margaret had passed away a few years before from a combination of heart failure and chronic obstructive pulmonary disease (COPD); she had spent the penultimate weeks of her life in hospital, and the last few days on a ventilator as her organs failed. She was unconscious until the point where the doctors finally admitted defeat and took her off the ventilator, after which she became quite lucid. In the hours that followed she talked with me and my sister but also seemed to be looking at something beyond us. She kept on saying, 'Oh beautiful, oh wonderful, oh joyous', and asked us, 'Is it real?' A little later she also cried out in joyful disbelief, 'Ma, oh Ma', and then seemed to speak to my father, saying 'Dan, oh my Dan, there you are', and finally, with a really radiant look on her face, she said: 'Jesus, Jesus, is that really you?' and then: 'Oh Jesus, yes, I'm coming.'

There's silence on the end of the phone. I let Martin ponder in the quiet before continuing. 'After this she became unconscious. My sister and I and another friend stayed by her bed. And then in the middle of the night when she was close to death, she said clearly: "Richard Dawkins was wrong. There is a God!" Those were her last words.'

Before I put the phone down, I tell Martin that I pray for him every day, and I ask him if he would like me to include him on the list of people prayed for at our church. Given his unwillingness to admit illness, I expect him to refuse but he says he would be grateful.

Then comes the awful news that the cancer has spread to his liver and his pancreas. His condition is now terminal, and the oncologist predicts that he has only between three and six months left to live. I drive down to their house expecting to find Martin in pieces, but he remains characteristically sanguine and speaks of the prognosis like a minor inconvenience. However, the strain on my friend's face is painful to see – her husband's policy of denial lending a surreal potency to the whole situation. Back at home, I continue to pray for healing from the cancer that now seems to be taking over his body, but I also ask God to make himself known to Martin and pray that he might experience a sense of his presence.

Martin is still on my mind as we head back to the hospital for the results of my own multitude of scans. It's a beautiful spring day and, as we drive through the rural landscape and into the outskirts of the city, I feel as if I am on an outing. The months of lockdown have begun to induce a lurking feeling of claustrophobia in much of the population, particularly those, like me, who are deemed clinically vulnerable. Hospital appointments provide one of the few excuses I have to get out of the house; so, as we navigate our way through the daffodil-dotted hedgerows and sunlight-drenched fields, I feel an incongruous holiday-like gaiety. The whole world feels full of light.

As we enter the surgeon's office, she begins by saying: 'First of all the good news.' Apparently, the CT scan and the bone scan have revealed no further malignancies in my body. I feel a surge of optimism, until I realize that there must be more. 'And the bad news?'

After what seems like an age, she responds. 'The MRI scan has revealed that there are indeed three areas of cancer in the outer and inner breast.'

I take a sharp intake of breath.

'They are a little bigger than previously but we don't need to be alarmed. But we do need to get a biopsy of the third tumour.'

Over the past few weeks of waiting, while time had seemed to have ground to a halt, the cancer had still been hard at work and continuing to grow. Time, it seems, is of the essence, and now I just want to get the tests out of the way and move towards a treatment as fast as possible. It also dawns on me that with this amount of cancer, a lumpectomy is no longer an option.

Then the surgeon drops the final bombshell: 'The tests also show that the cancer is HER2 [a more aggressive form of the cancer] so you'll be having chemotherapy before surgery. I'm going to refer you to an oncologist and we'll probably be looking at seven or eight cycles over six months.'

My heart sinks and, as the surgeon goes on to talk about options for reconstruction using natural tissue without an implant, I'm unable to concentrate on what she is saying: 'And as it's HER2 we will also be looking at bio-targeted treatments with the chemotherapy and for around twelve months afterwards.'

Increasingly alarmed, I try to calculate. Even when I had stage IV cancer, the treatment had only lasted for eight months, but when I add together six months of chemotherapy and twelve months of bio-targeted treatments a wave of despondency breaks over me – eighteen months of treatment! At the same time, I'm stung by a pang of shame. How can I be so ungrateful? I am so lucky to have access to these treatments – yet I can't help but feel daunted by the journey ahead of me.

Then, just when I think that the meeting is over, the surgeon adds: 'And as you have now had two types of breast cancer, I am going to refer you to genetics to have a BRCA gene test. If this comes back positive, I would recommend a double mastectomy.'

My thoughts immediately shoot to my children, and I realize that if there is a genetic cause it will, of course, have the additional impact of making them wonder about their own futures. Finally, she leans over, and she says with a disturbing tone of compassion: 'There's something else that I have to tell you. In the MRI scan the lymph nodes look big, so when we do the surgery we will also need to do a sentinel node biopsy to check if there is any spread.'

I feel like a diner gorged to the point where they cannot digest their meal.

As we emerge from her office, I look up and see that the sun is now obscured behind a thick blanket of grey cloud. I won't be sharing this news with Martin.

8

Hope

Hope is a strange and persistent beast. It rises in our hearts against all odds and clings to us even when evidence points to a situation as being beyond all hope. Martin Luther King Jr wrote from his Alabama prison cell that, 'Out of the mountain of despair comes the stone of hope.' We can find hope even in the worst circumstances of our lives. Hope enables us to envisage a future which is brighter than the present but also to experience the beauty of the here and now; to be able to live in the moment and to recognize that even when we are in the midst of pain and suffering there is still a reason for hope . . . and that reason is Christ.

In the Old Testament, the hope that the Israelites clung on to was that of a Messiah who would end their oppression and restore his kingdom on earth, and that hope came to them incarnate in the person of Jesus. This God-man taught extraordinary lessons of hope, speaking about a new kingdom, creation and age that would come and, as he talked and walked the dusty roads of Palestine, the irresistible power of hope broke through the dimensional barriers between heaven and earth. Hope was evident in everything Jesus did; from his sheer kindness and compassion which brought hope, to his miracles which were manifestations of God's hope breaking through into the world. Through his utter selflessness, he gave us hope that we could overcome sickness and death.

Today, against all odds, this hope can persist doggedly in the depths of our souls; not only the hope of life beyond death but also for life here on earth – even when this flies in the face of a cancer prognosis. Sometimes, clinging to hope can seem utterly irrational, but the Bible tells us that:

> Those who hope in the LORD
>> will renew their strength.
> They will soar on wings like eagles;
>> they will run and not grow weary,
>> they will walk and not be faint.
>
> Isaiah 40:31

This is the hope that I now cling on to. The landscape that I am moving through has shifted, but this seems to be an inevitable part of the cancer journey. Scientists have made enormous leaps and bounds in terms of understanding cancer's modus operandi, but this condition is mercurial and still has the potential to catch the medical profession off guard. Medics I have spoken to say that they still don't understand why cancer takes such radically different courses in people who are of the same age, gender and medical profile; why someone like me survived my initial stage IV cancer, while others lose their lives.

Cancer is an unpredictable foe and every new piece of information about the enemy has the potential to alter your trajectory. I try to prepare myself by thinking through the various scenarios that may unfold but always seem to be thrown off balance by new information. With my natural tendency to rush to conclusions, I had rather naively imagined a scenario in which, after surgery and a few weeks of radiotherapy, I would be able to pick up the reins of my life again. Instead, I'm facing eighteen months of treatment for an aggressive cancer that may have already begun to work its way around my system.

By now I should have learnt to live with the unpredictability, but I am still not prepared for the next twist in the road which comes in the form of a phone call from my surgeon, who informs me that the third tumour is yet another kind of cancer: this time the tumour is not only HER2 positive but also oestrogen receptor positive. This means that not only have I managed to get three different types of cancer but it's also possible that this is a recurrence of the previous cancer that has mutated. I ask tentatively if this new information has changed my prognosis and her answer is guarded: 'We have the right treatment plan, but we will need to treat this with respect.'

I query what this means in terms of surgery, and whether it now makes sense for me to have a double mastectomy as a preventative measure, to which she replies: 'Well, the breast tissue is certainly unstable. We'll have to see how you cope with the chemotherapy.'

I put the phone down, map out the terrain in my mind, and realize that I can no longer reassure myself that this is a new primary cancer and therefore unlikely to spread anywhere else. We seem to have come a long way in just a few weeks: from an initial plan for a single mastectomy for a primary cancer followed by a few doses of radiotherapy, to eighteen months of treatment for a cancer that may be more advanced. The irony isn't lost on me that, if I hadn't struggled with the idea of a single mastectomy, then it is unlikely I would have had the MRI scan to investigate the third area of tissue, let alone a biopsy that revealed the full complexity of my situation. God, it seems, really does work in mysterious ways. I feel profoundly grateful to my surgeon and the various NHS teams for the thoroughness of their investigation, and I am still holding on to God's promise that he will give me hope and a future, but at the same time can't help feeling rather daunted by what lies ahead.

As Easter approaches, there is a merciful hiatus in the relentless round of tests and consultations. On Good Friday, the family gathers for the rather messy business of dyeing eggs, one of the Lithuanian traditions (along with the Christmas Eve feast of herring known as Kucios) that have worked their way into the fabric of our family life. Then on Easter Sunday we gather around the family table and, before tucking into roast goose, engage in the traditional Lithuanian battle of the eggs. Everyone around the table takes a dyed egg and bashes it against their neighbour's. The one whose egg doesn't crack then engages their next opponent, and the champion egg is the one that emerges intact from the fray. It's great fun and a joy-filled interlude of normality and continuity.

A few days later I have my first meeting with the oncologist who will accompany me on this journey. Sitting nervously in reception, I am relieved to be greeted by another familiar face – that of the breast-care nurse who had managed all my check-ups after my last round of cancer. She smiles broadly and tells me how it is lovely to see me, and then – as if she has suddenly remembered the reason for my visit – tells me how sorry she is that I am back here again. When she introduces me to the oncologist as 'a trooper', I am strangely touched.

I warm to the consultant oncologist immediately – a delightfully erudite and slightly idiosyncratic man in whom I feel immediate trust (perhaps it is because some of my nearest and dearest have been prone to eccentricities that his rather offbeat humour fills me with confidence). He patiently takes me step by step through the treatment plan, which initially includes seven chemotherapy sessions starting at the end of April. For the first three sessions I will be given a combination of two drugs – epirubicin and cyclophosphamide – generally referred to as EC. This will be followed by four doses of docetaxel, the drug that worked so well on me previously.

After the third chemo cycle, I will also be given two additional monoclonal antibody treatments, pertuzumab and trastuzumab – which are designed to specifically target the HER2 protein on cancer cells; an example of the extraordinary developments in cancer treatments over the past few years. The only downside is that one of the drugs can negatively impact the way your heart works, so I will also have quarterly echocardiograms to ensure that my heart is still fully functioning. As all these drugs can also cause neutropenia (low neutrophil count) and leave patients vulnerable to infections, the treatments will be given on a three-weekly basis, in order to give my white cells time to reassert themselves before the next onslaught.

The oncologist tells me that my appreciation for straight talking precedes me and he doesn't hold back on the realities of chemotherapy, running through a terrifying list of potential side effects which range from the familiar baldness of cancer patients, nausea and fatigue, through to blood clots and the risk of life-threatening neutropenic sepsis. As the treatments suppress the immune system's ability to fight off infection, I am also told to avoid eating unpasteurized cheese, raw meat and uncooked eggs, which are rife with potentially harmful bacteria, for the duration of the treatment – as well as swimming. When I point out that one of my main leisure pastimes is wild swimming in lakes and rivers, as well as paddleboard-ing, his eyes nearly start out of his head.

'Absolutely not. No rivers, no lakes,' he tells me emphati-cally, waving an agitated finger in my face.

I come away from the meeting armed with copious amounts of paperwork outlining the worst that chemotherapy has to offer. I tell myself that this kind of litany is almost obligatory now as a form of legal protection for the medical profession. I'm holding on to the hope that I will emerge from the fray intact like a champion Easter egg. What the meeting has made clear, however, is that my world is about to be closed down even more effectively by cancer than it has been by Covid. Even before this diagnosis, I was regarded as clinically vulner-able as I suffer from asthma, bronchiectasis, and scarred lungs as a result of previous radiotherapy. So, even as the very strict-est Covid restrictions begin to ease, my contact with those outside my immediate family has remained pretty limited. But with the forthcoming treatment, I am soon to be elevated to the 'clinically *extremely* vulnerable' category, which will ef-fectively close my door on the world for the foreseeable future.

However, before I have to begin 'shielding', I have just over two weeks' grace, and I'm determined to take full advantage of this window of opportunity. So, I buy in large amounts of camembert and manage to sneak in one last session of pad-dleboarding on a nearby lake. As John and I glide together over the mirror-like surface of the water, watching miniature tiger-striped minnow dart amongst a forest of swaying emer-ald pondweed, I feel a sense of utter well-being that belies the reality of my situation. In the months to come, I will treasure these stolen moments.

9

Doors

With just a couple of weeks to go until I start chemotherapy, I realize that I also need to look at how the treatment will affect my work. My professional life has changed radically over the past few years; in 2014, when I was first diagnosed with cancer, I was working as Chief Communications Officer for World Vision and spending about a third of my time overseas, bouncing along dirt tracks in remote regions of sub-Saharan Africa or threading my way through the labyrinthine slums of South Asia. For six years, I had hopped on and off planes like buses until I no longer registered the oddity of a life spent in airports.

When cancer first stopped me in my tracks, my employer provided tremendous practical support and the staff collectively prayed for me, which I was so moved by; but, even in remission, it quickly became clear that I could no longer live this globetrotting lifestyle. I struggled with work for a few months until a fourteen-hour flight to Bogota, Colombia, brought home the impracticality of my situation. I boarded the plane at Heathrow full of anticipation, but by the time I got off at the other end I was so weak that I had to be taken through passport control in a wheelchair. So, a couple of months later, when the organization announced a management reshuffle, I took this as a sign that God had other paths for me to follow, and gratefully accepted redundancy.

While going through this first round of cancer, I was repeatedly given a wonderful piece of Scripture from Psalm 118: 'I shall not die, but live, and declare the works of the LORD' (v. 17 KJV). While I fought for my life, I hung on to that scripture like a life raft and, on the day I was told that I was in remission, I knelt before God and solemnly committed to him the life that he had given back to me. He had fulfilled his promise; now it was my turn, and I made it the mission of my restored life to 'declare the works of the Lord'.

At first, I thought that meant being ordained in the church. I wanted to make the biggest commitment possible to demonstrate my gratitude and would probably have joined a convent if I could; but, as I obviously couldn't be a nun, I decided that the most serious step that I could take was to be a priest. So, filled with zealous gratitude, I began a process of vocational discernment with the Church of England. I met with a vocational advisor, who rapidly discerned the depth of my calling and recommended me to the Diocesan Director of Ordinands (DDO) as a potential candidate for training, but God had other plans.

When I was first diagnosed with cancer, I was ironically given time to reflect that I had often denied myself with my relentlessly active life. Looking back, I began to see for the first time how God had always been there as a presence in my life, guiding my trajectory with his unseen hand. From my early childhood belief in the unseen to my rebellion years, and from my first tentative steps back to him to the blossoming of my faith, I began to see how he had spoken into and guided my life through Scripture, circumstances, encounters, and a series of inexplicable synchronicities or God-incidences.

Albert Einstein once said that there are only two ways to live your life: as if nothing was a miracle and as if everything is a miracle. Increasingly, in today's secular society there is too much of a tendency towards the former: a relentlessly atheist world view that leaves little room for the miraculous, sacrificing on the altar of rationalism the sublime possibility of a divine loving Creator with a plan for humanity. According to this logic, if something cannot be labelled or quantified then it cannot exist, and as God can't be bottled and categorized he therefore cannot exist, let alone intervene in human affairs. But, as I looked back over my life, I began to see a pattern in the random occurrences over the years; how for every challenge that I faced there had also been a blessing, as well as examples of small everyday miracles, such as the finding of that which I had believed lost, the piece of information that came to me just when I most needed it, or the message from a friend that seemed to speak into my deepest needs – needs that had hitherto been revealed only to God. Rationally it would be easy to explain these away as serendipity, but I was able to see how each incident was pregnant with meaning, and I began to understand that these everyday miracles were examples of God's grace breaking through into the world.

Faced with the initial stage IV cancer diagnosis, and the prospect of time potentially running out, I had felt an urgent need to communicate all this to my family. I started to put together photograph albums for my children, but soon realized that these only showed the events, places and people that figured in my life and said nothing about how I saw the world, what I believed, and crucially how I had experienced God – for this I needed words. So, as I lay in bed ravaged by the effects of chemotherapy, I began to write. My plan was to simply ring-bind the pages and leave them as a legacy for my children, but when, against all odds, I survived, I shared the manuscript with a close friend who persuaded me that it was worthy of publication.

Finding a publisher wasn't a prospect I relished. My mother had been a bestselling author and I had witnessed first-hand how hard it was to get a literary agent or a publisher to even review a manuscript. So, like Gideon laying out a fleece in the hope of a sign from God, I decided to send the manuscript to just one publisher and, if there was no interest, I would take it as a sign that the book was only meant for the eyes of my family.

I bought myself a directory of publishers and, opening the book at the letter A, ran my eye down the first few entries until my attention was arrested by a company called Authentic Media. I could hardly believe my eyes: the company in question was a Christian publisher based just 15 miles from where I lived – and they specialized in inspirational biographies and autobiographies. I could feel God's fingerprints all over my back but was still nervous about submitting my work to professional scrutiny.

When I had first written my story, I didn't think I'd be around to face the judgment of any who read it and, as such, had been very open about my feelings, particularly as I told the story of my journey through cancer. But once I had a life to go back to, I thought I might tone down some of the more raw and vulnerable sections of the book for the sake of my 'reputation'. However, the very next day I happened to mention to a colleague in World Vision that I had written my story and was thinking about trying to find a publisher and he immediately responded: 'I know exactly who you should send it to. I have a friend who is the head of a Christian publishing company. It's called Authentic Media. I'll get in contact with him.' I could hardly believe what I was hearing.

I was about to ask my colleague to hold off to give me some time for a final edit but, before I could stop him, he had fired off an email telling his friend that he must look at this manuscript, and only a few days later I received an email from Authentic Media asking to see the draft immediately. I was horrified as I didn't feel that it was ready for public consumption, but it felt as if God had opened a door for me and I realized that if I was to be true to my mission to 'declare the works of the Lord', then I had to be bold and to step through it. So, I wrote up a synopsis which I put in the post together with some sample chapters . . . and then waited.

Over the years I have often been amazed by the way in which some doors to opportunity have just seemed to open up before me, while at other times when I have tried to go down a certain path, the way has remained blocked, no matter how much I tried to force my way through. Some might put such opening of doors down to good luck or just being in the right place at the right time, but the writers of the Bible attributed this kind of supernatural doorkeeper intervention to the Holy Spirit. For example, Luke, the writer of Acts, recounts a time when the apostle Paul and his companions 'travelled throughout the region of Phrygia and Galatia, having been kept by the Holy Spirit from preaching the word in the province of Asia. When they came to the border of Mysia, they tried to enter Bithynia, but the Spirit of Jesus would not allow them to' (Acts 16:6–7). It isn't clear exactly how Paul and company were stopped in their tracks, but Luke records how they were then directed through a dream to travel instead to Macedonia, a move that ultimately led to the spread of Christianity beyond Asia into Europe and the western world. *This* was the door that God was directing them to walk through.

So, trusting in the divine Doorkeeper, I waited in anticipation, but when a couple of months went by with no word I began to question whether, like many times before, I was pushing at the wrong door. I was disappointed as I would have liked to follow in my mother's footsteps and become an author, but after a while I resigned myself to the fact that publication was not a path that God wanted me to go down. A small part of me was actually relieved because at least I didn't have to face the scrutiny of a publisher, or the public, and could simply print out copies for the kids; but, just as I was coming to terms with the rejection, I received an email from the new head of the publishing company. She had recently taken over, found my synopsis, and wanted me to resend the full manuscript immediately for review. I took a deep breath and threw caution to the wind. Twenty-four hours later, I received an email from the publishing company raving about my manuscript. Apparently one of the editors had taken it home to review the evening before and had not been able to put it down until she'd finished it. My life was about to change.

My memoir *Sea Changed* was published a year after my treatment ended and for a while went on to become a best-selling biography (and to my amazement was also nominated as Christian Resources Together's 2017 Christian Biography of the Year). Suddenly I was immersed in a whole new world of book signings, literary festivals and author events. I was invited to speak at churches and to groups all over the UK – and as far afield as Australia – about my story, and many who came to hear me speak would then take me to one side and share their own remarkable journeys.

My publisher also organized a whole raft of media interviews. As a magazine editor I had been a regular commentator on BBC, ITV, Channel 4 and Sky News and later, while working for World Vision, had spoken to the media about terrible disasters such as the Haiti earthquake and Japanese tsunami. But as an author I was now required to bare my soul in front of the camera and talk about my own story. Initially I found it an uncomfortable experience, but after a while I began to receive letters from viewers and listeners who talked about how much my story and book had helped them to understand that the surest path to God isn't always a straight line, and how he could be found in the most unexpected places – even a cancer diagnosis. I realized that this too was part of my commission to 'declare the works of the Lord'.

Then one day I was invited to do an interview with the Christian TV channel TBN that goes out on Sky and Freeview. I drove down to their impressive TV studios in north-west London, and was starstruck to discover that the legendary Christian writer and speaker R.T. Kendall was also in the building and that the previous interviewee was Philip Yancey. On arrival, I was guided into a vast auditorium with rows of empty theatre-style seats and a wide stage with a backdrop of a glittering cityscape (mercifully the interview was pre-recorded rather than live in front of an audience). The interviewer, Leon Schoeman, greeted me and settled me into a chair under the glare of several spotlights and, just before the cameras rolled, mentioned that the interview would be thirty minutes long. *Thirty minutes! Most of the news items I had done before had been a maximum of three minutes!* But then I began to talk and time lost its terror.

My interviewer seemed completely absorbed as I talked about how I had experienced God during my first cancer journey and, as the interview came to a close, he asked me to pray for those watching who might be treading the same path. And as I closed my eyes and opened my mouth, a prayer rose up from somewhere deep inside of me as if the Holy Spirit were speaking through me. Then, as we took off our mikes, Leon turned to me and enthused: 'That was truly terrific. I think God has something really important to say through you . . . I think I need to give you your own show!' Once again, I couldn't believe what I was hearing: if anyone had told me that, as a result of a cancer diagnosis, I would become a television presenter at the age of 53 (well past the 'sell-by date' for most TV channels), I'd have thought the idea preposterous.

Within twelve months, the first series of my new TV show, *Living a Transformed Life*, went on air. The show was a combination of my reflections on how God uses all the circumstances of our lives – even the most challenging – to transform us, and interviews with a succession of inspirational cancer survivors, pastors and healers about their stories and experiences of being transformed. At the suggestion of my publisher, I also wrote an accompanying reflection guide entitled *Sea Changed: A Companion Guide (Living a Transformed Life)*, and by the time I began work on my third book, *Soul's Scribe* – a guide to understanding and sharing your soul story – I began to feel like a real author. I even went so far as to launch an online course, 'Write Your Soul Story', for those who wanted to go down the path of also writing their autobiography or memoir.

I had soon realized, however, that being a Christian author wasn't going to pay the bills and, having lost my senior executive salary, I still needed to keep a roof over our heads. When I initially went to work at World Vision, my husband had given up work to look after the children while I jetted my way around the globe and back. Like Arnold Schwarzenegger's character in the film *Kindergarten Cop*, he'd proved a natural and had since trained and started work in primary education, but I remained the main breadwinner. Perhaps unwisely, I had embraced redundancy without a plan for how to replace the income, but within a few weeks of leaving World Vision I received a call out of the blue from my bishop asking if I could help him with a new strategy for the diocese. This convinced me that God wanted me to stay the course and was going to provide the necessary resources, and, once I stopped worrying and started trusting, the doors just kept on opening as an increasing number of Christian organizations asked me to help them with their brand and communication strategies. It was remarkable how I simply found myself, time and again, in conversation with the right person at the right time about the right opportunity.

However, despite the remarkable opportunities that God had brought my way, I still clung to the notion that all of this was a distraction and that my core calling was to ordination as a priest. And after two years of having deeply probing discussions with the DDO and writing lengthy essays on doctrinal issues, I was sent to a three-day residential interview known as a Bishop's Advisory Panel. Overseen by the impressive tower of Ely Cathedral and the watchful eyes of senior church leaders, I was quizzed on my theological biases and pastoral suitability and observed as I interacted with my fellow candidates. I found it a deeply challenging experience, but to my amazement I passed with flying colours and was recommended for three years of study at Ripon Theological College, which is located just outside Oxford.

Despite my love of writing, broadcasting and public speaking, I took the offer as a clear affirmation of my presumption that I should give all this up to commit to life as a parish priest. But no sooner had I reached this conclusion than I seemed to hit a number of bewildering but serious barriers involving the funding of my three years of study. Shocked by this unexpected turn of events, I was forced to consider whether in pursuing ordination I had actually been listening to my own guidance rather than God's. The crunch point came when I met up with a wise friend and mentor from my World Vision days, who seriously challenged me, saying: 'Kate, you are a strategist. God has given you all these opportunities to reach so many people with your message, but you want to give all this up and to spend only around ten per cent of your time doing what you are good at, namely communicating, and the rest of the time in PCC [parochial church council] meetings and worrying about the parish share. Do you really think this is God's strategy for your life?'

The logic was indisputable. I'd been so overwhelmed with gratitude to God for restoring my life that I was determined to stick to my earnest and heartfelt commitment to dedicate my life to him through ordination in the face of formidable evidence to the contrary. Now I was forced to accept that it might well be God who was closing the door on this particular ministry. I was terrified that the DDO would be furious with me for 'wasting' two years of her time but, when I rang her to break the bad news, she completely disarmed me by saying: 'It takes great courage to step off the train once it has started moving, but I think you are doing the right thing.' She actually helped me to see that I still had a ministry without a dog collar, 'declaring the works of the Lord' and helping others to do the same. However, now that ministry too seems to be grinding to a halt.

With treatment once again looming, I contact my long-suffering publisher to inform them that regrettably I need to cancel all the promotion for my newly launched title *Soul's Scribe*. The launch had taken place just two weeks before this latest cancer diagnosis, and I had planned a round of media interviews and speaking engagements, all of which I am now forced to abandon, along with my research trip for my next book. I also talk to TBN, who have just aired the second series of my show, to let them know that I won't be appearing on TV screens any time soon, and contact my clients to tell them that I need to temporarily wind down my brand and strategy consultancy.

As I deliver the news, I am overwhelmed by kindness as, one by one, people pray for me – one Roman Catholic charity I advise even arranging for mass to be said for me. Finally, I post a message on my website and social media platforms and am moved to tears by a torrent of messages of support and prayers. It's both humbling and comforting but, as I survey the landscape ahead, it feels as if there are now no discernible way-markers. My life has always been so purpose-filled; my calendar ever full of engagements; doors that seem to have been opened by God. Now it feels as if those doors are closing on me and I cannot help wondering: *Why is this happening to me? Where did I go wrong?*

I know that the Bible teaches that it isn't possible or necessary to earn God's love, salvation or healing; it is by grace we are saved, not actions, and faith and all that comes with it is a gift from God (Ephesians 2:8–9). Rationally, I also know that God doesn't *need* me to preach, write or broadcast his message (the idea that he is somehow reliant upon my puny efforts to 'declare the works of the Lord' is frankly ludicrous). I also don't believe that my recurrent cancer is the result of some kind of spiritual wrongdoing on my part. Habits such as smoking and overindulgence in alcohol which we sometimes think of as sinful have been shown to contribute to ill health, but the New Testament dismisses the idea, once widely held, that sickness is visited on us by God as some form of punishment (John 9:3). My head tells me that God's love is truly unconditional, and nothing we can do can separate us from the inexhaustible love of God (Romans 8:38–39), but my heart feels 'be-wildered'. Like the ancient Israelites I feel lost, wandering in a barren wilderness.

When God brought me through cancer the first time, everything had seemed so clear. I thought that I had been saved 'to declare the works of the Lord', and since then I've been driven by an overpowering sense of purpose. Filled with the Holy Spirit, I have boldly declared my faith, taken every opportunity to share my testimony of healing, and sought to come alongside others to encourage them in times of challenge. God has opened so many doors to remarkable opportunities and, by walking through them, I was convinced that I was fulfilling his mandate. But now I can only question why, once again, I have to walk this path of pain.

In my confusion I cry out to God, and in reply I'm reminded that wilderness times are not without purpose. In fact, it was during their wanderings in the harsh wilderness of the Sinai desert that God taught the Israelites his lessons for life, giving them the Ten Commandments and his rules for living under his lordship. Later on, after his baptism, Jesus was also driven into the wilderness, not because God was displeased with his Son but because he knew that these forty days of separation and solitude were an essential preparation for his earthly ministry. For Jesus, and for many after him such as the apostle Paul, the journey into the wilderness was seen as a necessary time of spiritual testing and discovery, and the barren desert was seen as a place of privacy and contemplation. It was a place of *being* rather than *doing*, where within the silence they were able to discover a new closeness with God. It was Isaiah who gave voice to God's great promise:

> See, I am doing a new thing!
>> Now it springs up; do you not perceive it?
> I am making a way in the wilderness
>> and streams in the wasteland.
>
> Isaiah 43:19 NIV 2011

A week before the treatment is due to commence, I join an online Encounter Prayer session with the Christian Healing Mission. As I close my eyes and slow my breath, I have the distinct impression that I'm hunched into a tightly curled ball, hugging my knees, my face buried and eyes tightly clenched like a distressed child. Lulled by the rhythm of my own breath, I gradually become still. Then, as my breath slows, I become aware of a presence, a figure standing before me that I recognize as Jesus. As I sit huddled on the ground, he crouches down and kisses me on the cheek. Then, standing, he places his hand on my head before pulling me forcibly to my feet.

I stand there rooted to the spot, but he propels me forward, pulling me with him, back through my memories.

Together we pass through the woodlands of my childhood and onto the streets of London; through fetid alleyways in the slums of Nairobi, and the corridors of the hospital where my youngest child was born; then along a familiar shoreline past ragged rockpools and towards a shallow estuary, the point where a stream meets the sea, until, together, we step into the water. As I move forward and the sea rises around me I begin to panic, and when I turn around to find my companion he is far from me, standing on a high rock. I cry out to him as the waters threaten to overwhelm me and, as the waves begin to break over my head, there is a single thought: 'When you pass through the waters, I will be with you' (Isaiah 43:2).

Part Two

The Voyage

10

Setting Sail

As the day of my first treatment dawns, I rise and go through my morning routine. I pray through the Church of England morning liturgy: 'The night has passed and the day lies open before us . . .'[1] and the psalm for the day – 'call upon me in the day of trouble; I will deliver you, and you will honour me' (Psalm 50:15) – words of such beauty, penned in the music room of pain. Then, bowing my head, I reach out to him: *O Lord and Father, I call on you. Deliver me once again from the scourge that is cancer. Lord, I trust in you. I know that you have plans to give me hope and a future, and today I lean into your promise that I will not die but will live and declare the works of the Lord.*

For the past few weeks, every step of this journey has seemed to take me into deeper waters and, as a passive recipient of ever more alarming medical revelations, I feel as though my world has been spiralling out of control. But with the commencement of treatment, it seems that we are moving into a new, more proactive phase and, no matter how much I may be dreading the thought of chemotherapy, there's also a sense of relief that the process of defusing the time bomb ticking in my body is getting under way.

Unfortunately, my husband's work commitments prevent him from being able to take me to my chemotherapy sessions.

The last time, I continued driving in-between treatments but managed to back into my neighbour's car; so, to prevent further risk to the public, my friend Maria offers to ferry me to and from the hospital. She arrives bright and early and sweeps me up in a wave of optimism and, as we speed through the morning sunlight with the car windows wound down and the radio turned up high, we sing our hearts out to 1980s soft rock, observed by fields of curious lambs. Then, on arrival, we pray together in the car park outside the local hospital's gleaming new cancer centre and, as I enter the portals of this temple of healing, I thank the Lord that I am being chauffeured by such a faith-filled friend.

The chemotherapy suite itself is a revelation. My initial meetings with consultants had all taken place in the outer courts of the cancer centre but, as treatment is now commencing, I'm finally taken into the inner sanctum: a large sweeping open-plan ward that curves around a central courtyard, the space divided into bays, each accommodating up to four patients in comfortable reclining chairs. The sun streams through floor-to-ceiling windows that look out over a garden bursting with daffodils and tulips below a vast azure sky. The overall impression of light is very far removed from my dismal expectations.

I'm one of the first patients of the day, and a cheerful male nurse guides me to a chair in one of the furthest bays where I settle myself down overlooking the garden. All is calm and I'm astonished by the ambience of peace and positivity. From this vantage point I am able to watch the chemo suite come to life, as the nurses clock on and one by one their charges arrive. Gradually the chairs in my bay are occupied. The seat in the corner is taken by a middle-aged man with the characteristic greying skin of a chemotherapy patient and a broad smile; beside me, an elderly gentleman waves and points at his throat to indicate that he is unable to speak, and the chair immediately opposite is taken by a tiny woman swathed in a vivid red shawl who introduces herself as the wife of a Methodist preacher and tells me that she has terminal oesophageal cancer. In the next bay, I spot a former colleague from World Vision UK surrounded by the paraphernalia of cancer treatment. I am used to seeing her in a work setting and her presence here seems incongruous. I abandon my post, walk round to her, and we sit together reminiscing until the cheerful nurse comes in search of his wandering charge and guides me back to begin treatment.

Once back in situ, the nurse approaches armed with a large cannula and my heart sinks. My long-term fear of needles has only been exacerbated by the fact that the previous round of chemotherapy has rendered my veins almost unusable. My left arm is off limits due to the lymphoedema that set in after the previous removal of my lymph nodes and, having been overused, the veins in my right arm are almost inaccessible.

These days medics must dig deep to obtain blood samples, so I've covered my right arm in industrial amounts of the kind of 'magic' numbing cream that is more commonly used by children, covering it with clingfilm to prevent it getting onto my clothes. The nurse's eyebrows rise as he peels back the plastic, unwrapping me like a chilled chicken, and as he begins digging in my cubital fossa (the inside of the elbow joint) I take a deep breath, clutch my cross and pray for an available vein – to no avail.

After several minutes of fruitless excavation, he moves on to my hand, but my veinous system appears to be missing in action. The numbing cream is providing little protection and, as a large black blood blister begins to form on the back of my hand, I have to apologize for an involuntary outburst of colourful language. Even armed with an ultrasound scanner, he cannot find a vein, and it dawns on me that if he really can't tap into my veins, the all-important chemotherapy won't go ahead. In desperation the nurse tries to heat up my hand and finally, after nearly an hour of digging, he manages to insert a line and the treatment begins.

As the cocktail of steroids, anti-emetics and chemotherapy gradually drip-feeds into my system, I gratefully accept the offer of tea and biscuits. Since my last bout of cancer, I have avoided anything vaguely pleasurable, such as alcohol, caffeine, red meat or sugar, but I now reason that the chemicals in my system are going to be more than a match for a couple of custard creams. I gaze around at my fellow patients, some of whom are so desperately ill that all they can do is sleep through the treatment that will, at best, buy them a few more weeks or months of life. But there is still an overwhelming air of peace about the place, the atmosphere reminding me of a retreat centre I once visited. We are a diverse and unlikely band of brothers and sisters, plucked from a myriad of different backgrounds with our varied histories, hopes and fears; fellow travellers brought together on this voyage by the common bond of cancer. As I look around at this unlikely community, I pray silently that the Holy Spirit will sweep through this place with healing in his wings and carry us all safely to shore.

After a couple of hours, my nurse reappears clutching two large syringes full of vivid red liquid which looks like the kind of substance you might find in a sorcerer's lair labelled 'poison'. He informs me that this alarming-looking concoction is cyclophosphamide, the C part of EC, and that I shouldn't be alarmed if my urine turns the same colour for a couple of days after it is administered. This part of the treatment has to be manually injected through the cannula and it is not a quick process, which gives me time to find out more about my ministering angel. He tells me that he comes from Zimbabwe, and we have an unlikely conversation about the state of the road between Bulawayo and Harare which I travelled in the course of my work with World Vision. Eventually he brings the conversation back to the subject of my treatment.

'We need to do something about your veins, as I don't think we can do this again.'

'Does this mean that I might not be able to have chemotherapy?' I ask, the timbre of my voice rising with anxiety.

'No, no, we will find an answer.' I really like this man.

It takes nearly half an hour to inject all of the 'witch's brew' into my arm and, after a further period of observation, I am free to go. As I get up to head to the door, my nurse presents me with a bright-yellow sharps container and a package of injections. He takes out an alarming-looking needle fixed to a spring-release system and tells me, 'Here's your G-CSF. You will need to inject these into your stomach once a day for the next six days.'

'What?! No one told me about this.'

The eyebrows rise again.

'What's it for?'

'It's to boost your white cell count and to protect you from infections,' he explains patiently.

Great – more needles. I have vague recollections of being given a single injection the day after chemotherapy treatment last time I went through this process, but this was administered by the nurses. Now it seems the responsibility has been passed to the patient, and a single injection has turned into six. This will be an interesting challenge given that I am incapable of watching anyone else injecting me without feeling sick and faint, but even I can see that I will have to do this – the last thing I want is neutropenic sepsis.

So, six hours after entering the chemo suite, I emerge into brilliant sunlight clutching my instruments of torture and find Maria sunbathing on one of the very few small patches of grass in the hospital grounds, her hair interlaced with daisies. We sit in the sun and talk about friendship and I tell her how grateful I am to have her in my life. I am on my way and, like my irrepressible friend, I am determined to make the most of the situation I find myself in.

11

Adrift

Since childhood I have been fascinated by the fantastical sub-conscious worlds that we inhabit while asleep. It's an interest that was fuelled by my father's obsession with the work of the psychotherapist Carl Jung and his theories on our dream states. From an early age I can remember being quizzed about my dreams over cornflakes by my father, who eagerly tried to interpret my subconscious wanderings.

Jung believed that, as spontaneous products of our uncon-scious, our dreams are the guiding words of our soul; the part of us that connects with God – an idea that also surfaces in the Bible. Dreams weave their way through the Scriptures: from Joseph's prophetic dreams of his own grandeur to the visions of the prophet Daniel, from the dream that sent Joseph and Mary into exile with their newborn son to the nightmare that spurred Pilate's wife to beg her husband not to take the life of Christ. Once these dreams were the preserve of prophets, but God also promised that 'your sons and daughters will proph-esy, your old men will dream dreams, your young men will see visions' (Joel 2:28) – a promise fulfilled at Pentecost when the Holy Spirit was poured out on all believers. Jung's interest in dream interpretation also has biblical precedents: Joseph and Daniel were both dream interpreters par excellence, predating the Swiss psychotherapist (and his nemesis, Freud) by a few thousand years.

Of course, not all our nocturnal symbols represent profound revelations from the Almighty, but over the years I have noticed that occasionally our dreams speak into our circumstances in uncanny ways. I can still vividly recall a dream that came to me in the months preceding my first cancer diagnosis. Every day, I was trying to simply work through the pain and fatigue, but one night I dreamt of a storm of apocalyptic proportions. As the wind whipped around me, I was handed a set of Tibetan handbells – believed by Jung to be a subconscious symbol for a warning or alarm. A short while later, I entered the storm of cancer.

Now once again I find that I am having vivid dreams. Perhaps it's the chemicals that course through my veins, or maybe something more profound, but on that first night after chemo treatment I dream of a young Indian guru, wearing a pale-russet kurta exquisitely embroidered with gold, who resembles Jesus. This Christ-like figure stands in a bright white room surrounded by praying women. Outside in a garden a line of people queue to see him, but before he allows them to enter he asks: 'Please wait while I pronounce this blessing.' Then, turning, he stretches out his hands towards me and says: 'May your arms be strong enough to swim, no matter how rough the waters.'

The first couple of days post-chemotherapy pass remarkably well except for my inability to administer my granulocyte-colony stimulating factor (G-CSF) injections. On day one, I muster up the courage but am unable to work the mechanism, and eventually my long-suffering husband takes me up to the hospital where they point out that it helps if you take the lid off the syringe! Red-faced, I return home and give it another go. Pinching a convenient roll of excess abdomen, I close my eyes and say 'one, two, three' before stabbing myself like an orange. Amazingly it works; the spring mechanism retracts the needle back into its case and I head downstairs to tell my husband, hoping for congratulations on my 'bravery'. Thank goodness I am not diabetic!

Aside from my embarrassment, I feel amazingly well and have extraordinary levels of energy despite little sleep. Chemotherapy patients are generally given steroids on the day prior to, and for two days after, chemotherapy in order to prevent vomiting. While very effective at controlling nausea, they also have the same impact as drinking around ten espressos – boosting your energy to almost manic levels and inducing insomnia. It's not a wonder that I feel well; I am on a medically induced high. A nesting instinct kicks in and I start tidying the house and making lists of chores to undertake during my sick leave.

Then, on day three, as the steroid-induced elation dissipates and the true impact of the noxious chemical cocktail begins to make itself felt, I wake to a body I hardly recognize. First light finds me like the victim of a shipwreck washed up on a strange shore. I am hardly able to move off the bed. It's as if every sinew of my body is shrieking, the very marrow of my bones aching, and I feel as though my body has been invaded by a foreign force. My mouth burns; my tongue is sticking to the roof of my mouth, which tastes rancid; my gums have developed an open sore. My digestive system feels as if it has been scoured with acid and, when I try to eat, every morsel of food seems to burn its way through my body. I try to ignore the underlying waves of nausea that keep threatening to bubble to the surface.

Even the air that I breathe tastes metallic and every sip of water like battery acid. I imagine that corrosive chemical substances emanate from every pore of my body and remember the indescribable miasma of chemotherapy – a distinctive smell that last time I tried to mask with a perfume whose scent I can no longer tolerate (the fragrance as well as the specialist shower gels and shampoos that I used during my last treatment were eventually consigned to the bin as even the vaguest exposure to the scent would trigger a gag reflex).

I lie alone in our converted attic bedroom listening to the sounds of the house coming to life: my husband harrying my youngest who is late for the school bus, the clatter of cups and tinny vocalizations of newscasters on the television, the thud of a closing door, wood on wood, the purr of a car engine and then . . . silence.

The day unfurls before me, empty and seemingly without purpose. The seconds, minutes and hours merge into one another, the only indicator of time being the rising and the setting of the sun. At lunchtime, I totter unsteadily downstairs, but by the time I reach the kitchen I have lost the desire to eat. I go back to bed and drift in and out of sleep until woken by the turning of a key in the lock that heralds the return of my husband and child.

I feel so blessed by their return – I know that so many people walk this road entirely alone – but I still feel alien, separated from them by an experience that, thankfully, they cannot share, and by the ever-present threat of Covid. In my ivory tower, I while away the daylight hours until the night comes, but not sleep.

In the small hours of the morning, I am visited by dark imaginings – what St John of the Cross called the 'dark night of the soul' – and I'm haunted by an unnerving sense of déjà vu, imagining that I never actually left this bed of sickness and the last six years of glorious remission were just an illusion. I tell myself that I must not give in to fears of the night and, instead, I must steel myself, strap on the armour of God, and stand in his strength against the marauding army of illness that threatens to engulf me. As daylight steals through the windows above my bed, I force myself to sit up and pray:

I arise today
through a mighty strength . . .

As the day progresses, I prop myself up in bed and read healing scriptures with gritty determination as if my life depended on them; but, as the days roll by, I become progressively weaker. My mind becomes confused – a chaotic whirlpool in which a myriad of thoughts swirl, collide, clash and merge – and my whole body seems to throb with disease, my heart pumping frantically in my chest.

I don't remember being quite this ill the last time I went through chemotherapy – in fact it was a blessed relief when the tumours began to shrink under the chemical onslaught and the pain receded – but perhaps it is just my memory playing tricks on me. Granted, I am seven years older and this is the second round of chemotherapy, but I hardly recognize the sorry excuse for a human that I have become, marooned on this island of illness. She is such a contrast to the woman who, only two weeks ago, crossed an entire lake on a paddleboard, gliding over the surface of the water like a swan. Now, mired in this chemically induced inertia, my body has transformed into something poisoned and broken. Although I know that the poison is administered for my own good – that cells must die so that I might live – I still find it a strange and radical transformation.

I attempt to read but the words won't stay still on the page. Instead, I try to listen to healing scriptures; to bathe in them, allowing them to wash over me in waves of hope; but I find I can't bear the voice of the narrator which seems to grate against my very bones.
I try to pray but the words won't come.
My spirit groans within me.
Weariness works its way through every fibre of my body.
My soul aches with the sheer effort of consciousness . . .
Slowly but surely, I give up the fight,
and slip away from the shore,
until I am adrift in deep waters.
Exhausted by the sheer effort of keeping myself afloat,
my strength ebbs away on the tide, and I begin to sink
down through the aquamarine depths;
away from the light playing across the surface of the waters.
I no longer have the strength to reach for the surface
and something inside of me tells me to 'let go' . . . and I fall
descending through the deep darkness,
the weight of water crushing down until . . .
sweet oblivion.
And there in the silent depths I wait.

In the last hours of May Day, John takes me to the hospital with a raging temperature. I am weak and confused, so he takes control and marches ahead of me into Accident and Emergency (A&E) like a herald, waving my lanyard that states in bold print: 'I am a patient on chemotherapy'. He is then sent back to sit in his car in the parking lot as I am rapidly taken through and parked in a cubicle. I begin to drift again but am awakened by a tussle taking place in the next bay between an injured and very vocal drunk, who is refusing treatment, and his remarkably patient police handlers. All that separates us is the thin blue line of the medical curtain.

Within minutes, however, I am the centre of attention as a doctor examines me, a nurse hooks me up to an electro-cardiogram (ECG) monitor, another takes my 'obs', and an-other tries to get a cannula into my arm. My veins are turning out to be my nemesis on this journey, but eventually she tri-umphs, and disappears with a phial of my blood. Left alone, I enter the kind of bewildered limbo state reserved for long waits in A&E. I begin to drift into sleep until yanked back to consciousness by the movement of my gurney. I sail down a corridor and am parked up in a small, brightly lit side room; my elevation to 'clinically *extremely* vulnerable' is now appar-ently complete and I have to be kept away from any potential infections.

In the early hours of the morning the doctor returns, jar-ring me back to consciousness, and informs me that I have a neutrophil count of zero and significantly raised infection markers. I once again have potentially life-threatening neutro-penic sepsis, a side effect of chemotherapy which can lead to organ failure. As I am hooked up to an intravenous line (IV) of antibiotics, I call my husband, who has fallen asleep in the car park, and tell him the news. Alarm bells ring when they tell me he can come to see me before I'm admitted, as one of the most distressing aspects of the pandemic has been that so many have suffered and died in hospital without their rela-tives being able to see them. He comes to my side, pale-faced and drawn, and my heart aches for him. Before I am admit-ted, I muster my last remaining resources, hold his hand and

encourage him, saying: 'God will bring me through this too.'
I'm aware of the seriousness of the situation, but something
in the core of my being is telling me that this is not how my
story will end.

Once my husband leaves, and I'm taken from A&E, any
last vestiges of fighting spirit leave my body.

I am vaguely aware of being wheeled down through the lab-
yrinthine corridors of the hospital to the acute medical unit
(AMU) where I am placed in an isolation room.
And as the door closes, I once again descend.
Down through the waters, away from the light.
Slowly, gently,
until my limbs gently settle on the distant ocean floor.
Swaddled in the stillness of the deep,
enveloped in silence.
All conscious thought ebbs away on the tide.
I bathe in the stillness, and silence permeates my soul.
Lulled by the invisible rhythm of the depths,
time loses its meaning.
Dreams meld with reality
as I rest on the far seabed.
Until gradually, in that liminal space
I begin to sense something other.
The numinous.
A presence, vast and uncontained,
indefinable but tangible.
An encounter with something endless and eternal
there in the pressing water.
And together we wait in the silence,
rocked in the arms of the deep.

12

The Depths

I am forced to simply *be*.
Deep down on the ocean floor
beyond thought,
utterly still.
Surrendered to something ancient
beyond time.

All striving ceases.
I lie in his embrace . . .

Until
eventually
slowly
my broken limbs are
raised from the shadowed wilds of the seabed.
In unseen arms, I begin to ascend.
Up from the azure abyss,
towards the penetrating light.
Passing through cerulean undertows
until finally
I break through the white-tipped surface
into the light of day.

13

Light

I become aware of my surroundings gradually; a slow reveal of impressions. The pale-green waters of my mind giving way to a bed of cool, crisp whiteness. A clear liquid drips through a sharp pain in my wrist. My back is numb.

Gone is the stillness of the seabed and the softly filtered light of the ocean depths. I am surrounded by bland ochre walls; a butterfly transfer winging its way across the doorway into what I imagine is a bathroom. A large frosted window is open a fraction, providing a glimpse of a slate-grey sky. Clouds covering the sun. I feel as if I have been drawn back into a muted reality, one that somehow feels less real than the phantasm – that incandescence in the stillness beneath the waters.

I can hear the beat of my heart, the rhythmic thudding of the engine of my body, pumping life through my veins. I listen, lost in wonder at the mechanism of life working away within, hermetically concealed beneath my skin. It strikes me how often I have failed to appreciate the exquisite and complex construction of the human body. And I imagine my blood – the fluid of life – working its way along 60,000 miles of my arteries, veins and capillaries which, if laid end to end, could wrap around the globe two and a half times. All that wonder contained within our feeble bodies.

I try to sit up but am as weak as a newborn child. So, I lie back down and drift in and out of sleep. As I slip again from the shores of consciousness, I am haunted by a sense of loss, a strange yearning for the depths. It's as if I have held something precious in my arms which has now slipped my grasp. I ache for the presence that cradled me in the stillness of the deep. Alone I drift, hoping to find my way back.

The sound of a door opening draws me back to the surface and, as I open my eyes, a plastic-protected nursing assistant peers in at me and then enters the room.

'How are we feeling then?'

I try to respond but my tongue is dry as biltong.

'You've really been in the wars.'

I follow her with my eyes as she busily makes her way around the room. She's not a young woman, probably in her late fifties, with a brutal mousy bob.

Spotting an empty water jug on the bedside table she says, 'Bet you want some water, don't ya?'

I nod.

She returns with a jug of water and pours some into the kind of sippy cup I used to give my children as toddlers.

She chatters away as she potters around the bed, tidying. 'You're one of my first customers, you know. It's my first day of training.'

I lift the child's cup to my lips and take a sip of cool water. I feel the moisture returning to my mouth. I try out my voice.

'Training?'

'Yes, I'm training to be an associate student nurse.'

I am nonplussed. What on earth would make a late-middle-aged lady decide to train for one of the most challenging and under-appreciated roles in this country – in the middle of a pandemic? My throat hurts but I have to know, so croak, 'Why?'

She thinks for a moment and then says, 'Well, most of my life, really, I've been in caring roles. This and that. But I really wanted this, you know, before I take my pension.'

She tucks in the corner of the bed and adds, almost as an afterthought, 'I really want to do end-of-life care.'

My curiosity is piqued, and I rasp, 'Why end-of-life care?'

As I ask the question, she stops what she is doing and her body goes rigid like that of a startled bird. She turns and looks at me as if she is actually seeing me for the first time. Suddenly she sags against the end of the bed. Her face crumples behind her medical mask, and a cry of inarticulate guttural grief rises up from deep within her.

Every fibre of my being wants to offer her comfort, to hug her. But I can't seem to move.

I manage to whisper, 'This is really personal, isn't it?'

She doesn't answer but leans against the end of the bed, silently sobbing.

Then, after a few moments, she gathers herself, straightens her back and smooths down the plastic apron. And when her eyes meet mine again, they are brighter and she states: 'I just want to help people have dignity at the end.'

Then she leaves. I don't get to hear her story – that would have been an intrusion into her grief – but I have a sense that I am on holy ground.

14

Silence

In the third week following chemotherapy treatment my neutrophil count at last begins to rise and the infection markers to fall and, finally, I'm deemed well enough to return to the world. John comes to pick me up from the hospital and I notice how pale and tense he looks. The strain he is under is obvious despite his efforts to hide it behind jokes about my release from prison.

As I emerge from my isolation room, I am able to get my bearings for the first time. I now realize that I have been hidden away behind a door on the right-hand side of a corridor which leads on to a busy ward. In my solitude I have been shielded from the round-the-clock activity of the ward and my fellow patients, some of whose lives have been unravelling and some saved. It's only now that I catch a brief glimpse of their faces as we turn to leave. So many stories that I will never know.

Back at home I realize that something has changed. I am certainly not a pretty sight; my hair has started to come out in clumps and there are bald patches amongst the lank greyness. I resemble a Shakespearean witch, complete with pallid complexion and sunken eyes, and a large cold sore throbs its way from lip to chin, completing the lack of glamour. But the change is not just bodily.

Now that I am no longer working, I have more time to my-self than I am used to. Every moment of my life to date seems to have been filled with activity, but now the days stretch out ahead of me like a blank canvas. With no work to occupy me, I yearn for some structure to my day. Every morning, I try to get out of bed and participate in the morning chaos before my husband and teenager leave but, once the door slams behind them both, quiet descends. As I wander the empty house, the silence rings in my ears and I realize that I am used to living with almost constant background noise.

When I was working, I would often keep the TV or radio news running in the background as I worked, a constant un-dercurrent of woes filling the air. While doing housework, I would tidy, dust and vacuum to loud music, prancing round the house like a teenager at a disco or a demented domestic goddess. While out driving, I would turn up the radio to full blast and, when walking, I would listen to music, my steps driven forward by a relentless beat.

Music has been part of my life for as long as I can remem-ber. I have no musical talent of my own but have always ad-mired those who do. As a student I helped to book bands to play at the university and was involved in the London indie rock scene in the 1980s. And throughout my life I have loved to see bands play live and feel the bass tones reverberating throughout my body. These days my musical tastes are fairly eclectic and range from bands such as Imagine Dragons and Florence and the Machine, to Christian worship acts like Casting Crowns and Kari Jobe. Now, as I spend an increas-ing amount of time alone, I realize that I don't want to listen even to my favourite artists. There is something too intrusive about the music; it's as if the sound is an invader shattering the silence. Feeling the need to turn down the decibels, I turn instead to the haunting meditative chants of Taizé.

I first heard a recording of the exquisite simplicity of Taizé chants while on one of my retreats and immediately felt as if I had been transported back to the Middle Ages. As I sat in the retreat centre chapel surrounded by flickering candlelight, I was lulled into tranquillity by ancient melodies and imagined the sacred words echoing through the corridors of a medieval European abbey:

Laudate omnes gentes
Laudate Dominum
Laudate omnes gentes
Laudate Dominum[1]

Simple phrases in Latin, French, German and occasionally English, repeating until they seem to become a part of you. It didn't matter that the meaning was obscured by a strange tongue – I was mesmerized, and after the end of my first battle with cancer I travelled to the source of the music, the commune of Taizé, in the Saône-et-Loire Department of Burgundy in France. It is a sanctuary where brothers from different Christian traditions and more than thirty countries seek a new way of worshipping God that cuts across human differences and reaches into the heart of the soul.

I sat cross-legged on the floor of the minimalist chapel in Taizé, surrounded by a multicultural sea of people, all facing a simple altar dressed in white and pale green at the end of the hall. Behind the altar, streams of fire-red linen fanned out like the rays of the sun, the surface of the fabric alive with the flames of a multitude of candles. To the right, a large cruciform icon flickered, its gilded Christ illuminated by the flames. Every face in the room was bathed in fire and flame, the warmth punctuated by the white robes of the Taizé monks who filed into the hall and took their places kneeling among tie-dye and backpacks. As the voices of those present rose and fell like waves in words that transcend culture, I gave myself over to the moment. Worshippers undulated like saplings in the wind, swayed by the meditative power of the music, as the sung truths permeated each person – body, soul and spirit. I lost track of time and knew only that God had brought me to this place and, as I sang, I felt a new strength and healing rising up from the depths of my soul.

Now far from the South of France I spend hours lost again in the beauty of the ancient chants that seem to embody holiness; the rising and falling of voices joined in unity in praise of God – sounds symbolic of God's peace:

Bless the Lord, my soul
and bless God's holy name.
Bless the Lord, my soul
who leads me into life.[2]

However, after a few days even this glorious music feels like an intrusion into the silence. I start to seek the space between the sounds until all that is left are my footsteps echoing around the empty house and the rhythm of my own breath.

As I begin to recover, I go out into the garden and raise my face towards the early summer sun. Gazing into the vast expanse of sky, I watch a few stray wisps of cloud drift by. Beyond my sight, the sky grows darker until eventually all light is extinguished by the enormity of the universe, galaxy upon galaxy, worlds without end – the immeasurable breadth and depth of our reality. As I look up into the endless sky, I am awestruck by the paradox of the transcendent being, the creator of the stars, who took human form and walked on the face of the earth. The Alpha and Omega, the beginning and the end, who exists beyond time but is closer to me than my own skin; who knows my every thought, as I stand here battered and broken, revelling in his mystery.

In the quiet, I can feel him almost as tangibly as I did when I plunged into the depths. The air, like the water, is charged; tangible and alive with his immanence, unseen but omnipresent . . . *in him, we live and move and have our being* (Acts 17:28).

15

A Spacious Place

I decide that I need to take control of my physical disintegration. The last time I went through chemotherapy-induced hair loss, I was referred to a patient hair-care clinic housed in a local hairdresser's and barber's salon which my father had always favoured because it was owned by a Greek called Christo. Over the intervening years I'd become very friendly with his daughter-in-law who, inspired by my story, had been recommending my book *Sea Changed* to her clients. So, it's with some trepidation that I call to tell her that I once again require her services.

A consummate professional, she responds without missing a beat, saying: 'I'll come over to you.' There's no hint of pity, for which I am grateful – the last thing I want is sympathy. She arrives later the same day, covered from head to toe in personal protective equipment (PPE) and armed with scissors and hair clippers. 'At least you don't have all that long hair now,' she says as she tackles what remains of my grey crop. Less than half an hour later, I am shorn. Looking at myself in the hand mirror, it strikes me that I now resemble the bald-headed character Uncle Fester from the children's film *The Addams Family*, but as I run my hand over the slight remaining stubble the sensation is liberating. I am no longer falling apart follicle by follicle, which makes it easier to come to terms with this new normality.

As my next cycle of chemotherapy looms, I'm advised that something has to be done about my veins and my oncologist recommends the insertion of a Porta Cath, a device that is used to give treatments. I am familiar with the procedure, whereby a 'port' is implanted under the skin of your chest and attached to a thin flexible tube that is threaded into a large vein above the heart. Each time you are given chemotherapy, a needle is inserted through the skin and into the port. The last time I went through chemotherapy I came to think of this 'tap' into my veinous network as my best friend, so I agree willingly. However, when I am given a slot the day before my next chemotherapy treatment, I realize that the nurse who next administers my chemotherapy will need to go in through a fresh surgical wound, which makes me feel rather squeamish.

At my pre-operative assessment, I'm greeted by a young radiology nurse who radiates confidence. She sits me down and, spotting the ever-present wooden cross in my hand, asks, 'Are you a believer?' I tell her that I am and the most extraordinary conversation ensues. She speaks passionately about her own Pentecostal faith and her firm belief in the relationship between faith and healing and, before I know it, I'm telling her the story of my previous healing from cancer and of the trust I continue to have in God. She breaks into passionate praise and, dispensing with all protocol, she takes my hand and we begin to pray, our words tumbling over each other's like rapids. With closed eyes I pray for her healing ministry as the hands and feet of God in this hospital, and she speaks wonderful sacred words of healing, prayers peppered with ancient Scripture and future hope. And once again God's promise comes to me as, completely unprompted, she prays: 'Lord, I know you have plans to prosper Kate, not to harm her, plans to give her hope and a future' (see Jeremiah 29:11).

As she speaks, I have the uncanny feeling that Jesus is standing over us – one hand on the shoulder of my prayerful medic and the other on mine – and that the Holy Spirit is moving within us and around us. It's as if the Spirit is washing over us like a great tidal wave of hope, and tears of joy run down my face. I've no idea how much time has passed by the time I open my eyes again and look into her radiant face. As she leaves the room to fetch the doctor who will perform the procedure, I simply raise my hands to the Lord and tell him 'You are amazing!'

When I return a couple of days later for the procedure, the prayerful nurse once again comes to greet me and, in the waiting area, we pray together – vocally and passionately. I'm not sure what the other patients make of us, but it feels absolutely right. As I wait, I take a couple of the diazepam tablets kindly dispensed by my GP. During my previous Porta Cath insertion, I was blissfully ignorant of the procedure, having been given general anaesthetic, and I reasoned that given my squeamishness about needles it would be easier for everyone concerned if I was slightly sedated. By the time my prayerful friend takes me into the operating theatre, I am feeling mercifully bleary.

On the operating table, my face is covered by a plastic tent and, as I am given the first injection of local anaesthetic, I feel a hand take mine and a familiar voice begins to narrate the procedure. As an incision is made in my neck, I feel no pain, only pressure, followed by a curious sensation as a flexible tube is fed into my superior vena cava until it reaches my upper chest area. As I've already had one Porta Cath removed there is some concern that my veins will be too damaged to insert another but, after some debate, my guardian angel informs me that all is going well. To which I could only reply, 'Praise the Lord.'

When the doctor tells me that he is about to dig a hole in my chest to insert the port, I feel my muscles tense up. But once again I feel a hand take mine and, clutching my wooden cross, I inwardly recite the words of one of my favourite psalms:

> Praise the LORD, O my soul;
>> all my inmost being, praise his holy name.
> Praise the LORD, O my soul,
>> and forget not all his benefits –
> who forgives all your sins
>> and heals all your diseases,
> who redeems your life from the pit
>> and crowns you with love and compassion,
> who satisfies your desires with good things
>> so that your youth is renewed like the eagle's.
>
> Psalm 103:1–5

I first became familiar with this psalm during my last cancer journey and, since going into remission, have turned to it frequently as a form of prayer, giving thanks for my deliverance. Now, as I mentally pore over the symbolism, the tension begins to fade away; it's amazing how praise seems to help you cope, even when someone is busy carving into your chest with a scalpel. Perhaps this is why Isaiah tells us that we must put on 'a garment of praise' (Isaiah 61:3); when we shift our focus from our own situation, fears or melancholy, to the awesome and boundless nature and love of the Almighty, our troubles seem to pale into insignificance. The whole procedure takes around two hours, during which I manage to stay stock still through a combination of Scripture, diazepam and the caring support of my prayerful friend.

The day before my second chemotherapy cycle, I join the Christian Healing Mission Encounter Prayer group on Zoom. We pray '*Abba*, Father' and, once again, we're invited to notice where Jesus is for us at this time. I feel the old scepticism rising but am taken by surprise by an overwhelming sense that I am once again on the seashore walking beside Jesus. At first, I walk in step with him, the waves lapping at my feet, but as we near an estuary I turn away from him and move deeper into the water. Facing the sun, I walk through the waves towards the horizon until once again the waters break over my head. Soon I am out of my depth. I struggle to keep afloat but the undertow claims me and I begin to sink down through the sun-dappled waters towards the shadowed depths.

Once again, I am descending to the ocean floor. A profound sense of peace draws me deeper, and I sense that I must let go and allow myself to fall. Until once more I settle on the shifting sand of the seabed, my heart stills, and there I wait.

All I am conscious of is my breath,

and the other,

that presence,

older than time.

I lie there safe,

filled with eager anticipation.

Until again

a ray of light penetrates the darkness,

and I begin my ascent.

I do not see him,

but I know that it is he who has reached down,

lifting me, up from the abyss.

Until breaking through the surf,

I rise higher and higher

above the sea line.
Through the sunlight
until together we stand on a high rock
towering above the pale-white shore below.
From here I gaze out
over the breathtaking beauty
of the cobalt-blue horizon,
where waters and sky meet.
Over the grass-knit sand dunes
to a wild land beyond.

A single line of Scripture repeats in my thoughts:
     'He has brought me into a spacious place,
     He has brought me into a spacious place.'

When the Zoom call is over, I google 'scripture, spacious place'
and find that the words come from Psalm 18, and as I read the
rest of the Scripture my breath is taken away:

The cords of death entangled me;
          the torrents of destruction overwhelmed me.
The cords of the grave coiled around me;
          the snares of death confronted me.
In my distress I called to the LORD;
          I cried to my God for help.
From his temple he heard my voice;
          my cry became before him, into his ears . . .

He reached down from on high and took hold of me;
          he drew me out of deep waters . . .
He brought me out into a spacious place . . .

                                        Psalm 18:4–19

16

Holy Ground

The next day, as I wander into the chemo suite, I'm greeted with a frown from the male nurse who had previously had the unenviable task of getting a cannula into me. I point to the dressing over my new Porta Cath and tell him, 'I've got a tap now', and he looks more confident. I still need to mentally gird my loins as he inserts a long needle through the fresh wound in my chest, but the whole procedure is over very quickly and the experience is considerably less gruelling than the last attempt to get chemotherapy into my veins. I give silent thanks for my Porta Cath.

I find a seat in one of the bays and, as I wait for the treatment, I look around me. The place is just as peaceful as I remember it, and as I register the faces full of hope, pain and sometimes despair it strikes me once again that I am on holy ground. As the preparatory cocktail of steroids and anti-emetics flows into my veins, I put on my headphones and open the Daily Office prayer app on my phone. I close my eyes and listen to the comforting familiarity of the liturgy, and follow along with the responses in a barely audible whisper. I'm conscious that I must appear to be talking to myself but hope that the cross and Bible on my side table might witness to the fact that I am actually praying and that my actions will add to the sense of positivity in the place. The bustle of the chemo suite fades away until I am conscious only of my heartbeat and the familiar words of Psalm 103: 'Bless the LORD, O my soul . . .'

Opening my eyes, I register the faces around me and pray for each of them, one by one. An elderly lady comes and sits in the chair opposite and a nurse pops her head round the corner and asks, 'How are we, girls?' (I rather like the idea that we are still girls.) Later on, a sound of clapping resounds along the bays as a patient rings the ward bell to signify the end of her cancer treatment. It's a joyful moment in which everyone participates, the nurses forming a corridor of applause as she makes her way out of the chemo ward for, hopefully, the last time.

As a nurse patiently infuses me with the bright-red EC con-coction, I comment on how upbeat the place feels and she replies, 'Yes, it's very strange. It's such a lovely atmosphere on this ward. It's why I love working here.' Her face is radiant, like that of an angel. As my veins fill, I watch in wonder as the other nurses move among the filtered sunbeams, dispens-ing hope, and for a moment I imagine Jesus moving among them – all caring and compassion.

My oncologist has wisely reduced the dosage of chemo-therapy in an attempt to prevent a repetition of the previous calamity, but on the third day post-treatment I once again be-gin the descent. Fatigue drags me down like a millstone, and the very marrow of my bones seems to ache. Mercifully, the nausea is more manageable, but it still feels as if the glorious flavours of life are no match for the chemicals in my blood. Chemotherapy seems to have engendered a type of synaesthe-sia, and some sights and colours now have their own flavour that disgusts. I feel suffused and surrounded by an atmosphere that is profoundly alien.

Yet something deep inside tells me that not all that whispers in my veins is of death. There is something else present, a positive power that is not of human will but of God. In his letter to the Romans, the apostle Paul wrote that 'the Spirit of him who raised Jesus from the dead is living in you' and that 'he who raised Christ from the dead will also give life to your mortal bodies through his Spirit, who lives in you' (Romans 8:11). This is the power that silently moved its way through the body of the Christ as he lay in his cold dark tomb, reversing the natural entropy and decay of the universe, bringing life where there was death. The Spirit of the Father, that great consciousness who exists beyond our limited time and space, had changed matter, resurrecting his beloved Son, building a bridge between our two realities. That same extraordinary power lies within us and, the Bible says, can also repair our damaged cells and broken bodies. The Greek word for 'to give life' in this passage from Romans is *zoopoieo*, which refers to the spiritual power to make alive, reanimate, restore to life, give increase of life, and reinvigorate something that is dead in your life or a body part that needs healing. When I close my eyes, I try to imagine the power of the Holy Spirit coursing through my veins, burning away the cancer. As I do so, I'm haunted by memories of deep waters and the connection with that divine presence I felt there.

At night I dream of the sea. In my sleep, I yearn to dive into crystal aquamarine waters but, before I am able to, I awake with a sense of loss. It only reinforces my conviction that I have experienced something profound – not just the outpourings of a delirious mind but something deeper. It's as if I have surrendered to something ancient and transcendent, which keeps drawing me back, and I feel a burning need to understand more about what I experienced and what this means for me.

I begin to pray and, as I reach out for meaning, answers start to find their way to me through different channels. A friend recommends a book to me called *Healing Words: The Power of Prayer and the Practice of Medicine* by American medic Larry Dossey MD. Dossey, who was chief of staff at a medical centre in Dallas, spent ten years examining available scientific evidence for a relationship between healing and prayer. He painstakingly reviewed a wide range of experiments – involving not only humans but everything from bacteria to fungi, red blood to plant seeds, as well as cancer cells in humans and mice – and finally came to the conclusion that prayer *is* able to directly impact the outcome of various conditions ranging from blood pressure to cancer, and to affect everything from haemoglobin levels to wound healing. He never goes so far as to claim that *all* prayer heals (and is at pains to point out that it's impossible to predict how a patient will respond) but he does claim that scientific studies show that prayer *can* and does heal – an idea that remains controversial in many quarters.[1]

In his book, Dossey quotes a study by Spindrift Research in Salem, Oregon, which looked at how the intention of prayer impacts healing. What the researchers found was that both *direct* prayers for a specific outcome – for example, for a certain treatment to be successful – and more *indirect* open-ended prayers of the 'Thy will be done' variety were effective, but that those prayers that didn't specify the outcome seemed to yield greater results.[2] As I read this, it dawns on me that throughout my previous cancer journey I had characteristically taken a very outcome-oriented approach to prayer. As I went through the different stages of my treatment, I had prayed for specific desired outcomes: that my scans would show the chemotherapy was working, that the surgeon would successfully remove all the remaining cancer, that the radiotherapy would help to buy me more time. It's an approach that is perfectly understandable (although we have to be careful not to end up telling God what to do), but what Dossey identifies is the power of 'prayerfulness [which] is accepting without being passive, is grateful without giving up'.[3]

Rather than going into 'battle' against the cancer, this approach seems to require us to say to God, 'Thy will be done', and really mean it. To pray like Charles de Foucauld: 'Father, I abandon myself into your hands; do with me what you will. Whatever you may do, I thank you. I am ready for all; I accept all'[4] – even when his will seems to be taking you to the border between life and death. It's not an easy task, as it requires us 'to stand in the mystery, to tolerate ambiguity and the unknown' and to honour 'the rightness of whatever happens, even cancer'.[5] It's about stopping the struggle to stay afloat and allowing oneself to be taken down into the depths, through the emerald waters, away from the light, to a place of silence and stillness, where there is no sense of time or space. To a liminal place where you are forced to simply be, surrendered and still, cradled by something ancient that existed before time, vast and unending, uncontained and eternal, magnificent and kind.

I share my reflections with a Christian friend who is also an expert in Jungian psychoanalysis and he recommends that I read a book by Bede Griffiths called *The Marriage of East and West*. Griffiths was a remarkable man, an Oxford-educated Benedictine monk who left England in 1955 and went to southern India in a bid to discover what he called 'the other half of his soul'. What he found there so moved him that he stayed and dedicated the rest of his life to exploring the relationship between the more 'intuitive' mysticism of the Indian subcontinent and western Christian thinking, founding monasteries and developing a monastic way of life that bridged the Christian and Hindu traditions.

Bede had come to the rather Jungian belief that there are two parts to our souls: one part that is masculine, conscious and rational which the Swiss psychoanalyst called the *animus*, and another part that is feminine, unconscious and intuitive which he called the *anima*. Bede believed that in the modern world a schism has developed between the two parts of our soul at an individual but also at a societal level. As he straddled two cultures, he was able to compare what he saw as masculine western rationalism with the intuitive approach of the East, and concluded that since the Middle Ages something has been lacking in both the western world and the church.

His argument was that today in the West, we are 'living from one half of our soul, from the conscious, rational level' and need to 'discover the other half, the unconscious intuitive dimension'[6] – an intuition that lies beneath our consciousness. He points to the fact that Christianity was originally a religion from the East, and argues that we in the West need to surrender our grasp on reason and reconnect ourselves to an intuitive consciousness; to learn to surrender ourselves to 'the deeper intuitions of the Spirit' that come 'from the presence of the Spirit in the depths of the soul'.[7]

As I read on, it's as if a door unlocks within me and I am visited by a series of memories. It's late at night and I'm sitting at the kitchen table at my childhood home, Larkland. My father sits opposite and is reading to me from Jung's *Memories,*

Dreams and Reflections about the psychoanalyst's search for his own 'anima', his intuitive unconscious.

He shares with me a few lines from a poem he is writing:

Anima is the spark
That lights
Or burns a way
Only the animus knows[8]

Another memory: I'm walking in the warm air of the golden afternoon sun with my friend Jayanth, beside the temple-strewn sea line of the southern Indian city of Chennai. We've just left the cool interior of the purported tomb of the apostle Thomas and are walking away from his whitewashed cathedral basilica which sparkles down by the shore. As we walk, Jayanth recounts the story of how Thomas left his doubts behind in Jerusalem and, long before Bede, made the journey to India to set up a school for Christians.

These 'Thomas Christians', who still worship today in the state of Kerala, wove together early Christian theology and the mystical beliefs of their homeland into a trinitarian faith in God, the Absolute Consciousness, who is Sat-Chit-Ananda: Existence, Consciousness and Bliss, and also God the Father (Sat), Son (Chit) and Holy Spirit (Ananda). According to this way of thinking, it's Jesus the Son who points the way to the God beyond and God within – an idea reflected in Jesus' own promise that if we 'abide' in him, he will in turn abide within us (John 15:4–5). But it's through the spiritual practice of meditation, more familiar in the East than in the West, that the Thomas Christians believe we can awaken this transformative 'inner Christ'.

Yet another scene surfaces from my memory. I'm perched cross-legged on a crimson cushion, my knees touching a polished wooden floor, my head swimming with the heady scent of incense. Beside me is a blonde-haired Swede in a sari and, to my right, a young bearded American. Through the window of the study centre I can see the fluttering multicoloured prayer flags of McLeod Ganj, the old district of the Himalayan town of Dharamsala, home to the exiled Tibetan Dalai Lama. Beyond are the snow-dressed peaks of the Dhauladhar mountain range of Himichal Pradesh. At the front of the room, a middle-aged monk gowned in deep maroon and yellow chants the dharma in sonorous tones and tells us to 'embrace the mantra'. I close my eyes, but my mind abounds with doubts, impressions and questions.

The intensity of these memories almost overwhelms me and I begin to get glimpses of connection: my father's pursuit of his unconscious, my friend's revelations on the shores of Chennai, the extraordinary draw I feel to the subcontinent of India with its colourful, chaotic brand of mysticism which seems to pervade every aspect of life.

I share these reflections with my spiritual director who, to my amazement, reveals that as a young man he had actually travelled to India in order to study under Bede Griffiths. So many synchronicities and connections. I feel a sense of anticipation, as if I am uncovering something deeply mysterious and precious. I know that I am on the track of something important and wonderful, and that I am being guided towards these truths. Despite my weakened state I desperately want to continue exploring, to feed the deep hunger inside of me that is driving me to learn more.

As I continue to read, I recognize that I am truly a product of the western world. Most of my life I have trusted in what my head told me rather than my heart. I have prized 'thinking' over 'feeling', and most of my life decisions have been reached through rationalism rather than intuition. This even extends to my faith; the reason why I turned my back on the church in my youth was because I couldn't reconcile the paradox of an all-loving God who could allow my father to suffer, and it was only through the wisdom of great thinkers like C.S. Lewis that I managed to find my way back to him again.

When I did return to the fold it was to the Anglican Church which balances the authorities of Scripture, tradition and *reason*, and over the past few years I have continued my theological studies in a bid to better understand my Creator and Saviour. If I am honest, I have always felt slightly uncomfortable with more overtly emotional expressions of faith, and distrustful of those whose faith seemed to be blind. Didn't God give us the ability to *rationalize* for a reason and didn't Jesus say, 'Love the Lord your God with all your heart and with all your soul and with all your *mind*' (Matthew 22:37, my italics)?

During my first cancer journey, as I looked back over my life and wrote my memoir *Sea Changed*, I had slowly come to realize how God also reveals himself to us through the experiences and circumstances of our lives, and how he continues to guide us through Scripture, encounters with others and God-incidences. I had even embraced the idea of the miraculous, which flies in the face of rationalism, but I still hadn't been able to completely let go of an underlying scepticism honed by my years as a journalist.

Occasionally I had touched on a more intuitive experience of Christ through Encounter Prayer, but in that hospital room I was exposed to something completely beyond my comprehension. I could rationalize away my 'ocean floor' experience as a product of a sepsis-ridden delirious mind, but something inside me has shifted. It feels as if a door has opened in my mind and that I am being beckoned through that doorway into an unfamiliar realm and I cannot ignore the summons. 'Deep calls to deep' (Psalm 42:7), and every atom of my being yearns for that connection I experienced in the depths of consciousness to the deity whose nature is far beyond our comprehension – the God whose thoughts are as far beyond our understanding as heaven is from our reach (Isaiah 55:9), whose love plumbs depths we cannot imagine.

As I read on, I am amazed to discover that in eastern spirituality, bodies of water represent 'the powers of the "unconscious", the elemental passions, which lie beneath the surface of conscious life'[9] (an idea that correlates with Jung's belief that dreams of oceans, lakes and rivers represent the part of us that lies beyond our waking reach) and, according to Griffiths, 'we have to die, to go under the waters of the unconscious, in order that we may be reborn and experience the power of a new life'.[10]

Is this why I long to descend to the depths once again, to surrender in the stillness and to simply be in the presence of the one who is unseen, unfathomable and eternal? Must I too let go of what I think I know of God, embrace the mystery and be willing to go beneath the waters of the unconscious in order to lie in his unseen arms once again?

17

Ancient Paths

A silver light creeps through the attic bedroom window, bright beams penetrating the darkness. I tiptoe down the stairs and out into the moonlit garden and gaze up at the sky. I remember a night like this in my childhood, when my father roused me from my bed and, together, we softly trod down the stairs, out through the cottage door and walked between the luminescence and the moon shadows.

I raise my face to the sky and bathe in the moonlight, before climbing the stairs again to watch the ethereal shadows dance across my quilted bed. As I finally slip into blessed sleep, my mind is free to roam and I dream that I am walking barefoot along a pale shell-scattered seashore, crushed carapace cutting into flesh. Bending down, I gather a handful of the sea-soaked earth, rocks of ages worn down into dust, so fragile that they are lifted by the breeze. Millions of grains, some gypsum white, others sandstone red, each infinitesimally small but with their own story to tell. Walking on I come upon a basking turtle, sunlight glinting off its dark-green armoured shell. I bend down and pick up the animal, and hold him to my chest, his gnarled old man's face smiling into mine.

A turtle is one of the most ancient creatures on our planet. Their form has not changed a great deal in the last 250 million years and they are one of the few animals alive today that bear any resemblance to the dinosaurs that roamed prehistoric Earth. They are ancient beyond our imagining and, according to Jung, when these primordial creatures populate our dreams, they represent the need to connect with something ancient that lies deep within ourselves.

I find a passage in the book of Jeremiah in which the prophet tells us to:

Stand at the crossroads and look;
        ask for the ancient paths,
ask where the good way is, and walk in it,
        and you will find rest for your souls.

                                                        Jeremiah 6:16

So, I go in search of ancient paths and a way of being and thinking from long ago. I soon realize that my quest is taking me into unfamiliar territory for many modern Christians and down some unorthodox avenues of exploration.

I begin by following Bede's advice and look back to a time before we lost that connection with the intuitive part of our soul – back to the history and experiences of the very first Christians who first sought to understand the meaning of Emmanuel ('God with us') and his teachings.

Two thousand years ago in Palestine there was little real understanding of the workings of the body, let alone the mind, and the idea of the consciousness – intuitive or otherwise – had yet to be formed. However, certain ancient accounts of Jesus' teachings do point to an awareness of God that goes beyond a rational understanding. In particular, there have been different interpretations of Jesus' assertion that 'the kingdom of God does not come with your careful observation . . . because the kingdom of God is within you' (Luke 17:21). Some modern thinkers believe that Jesus meant that the kingdom of God is within our hearts, others that the kingdom is in our midst in the person and presence of Christ, but both interpretations seem to point to an intuitive experience of God.

This is certainly how this statement was interpreted by the Gnostics, a group of second-century Jewish Christians whose name derived from the Greek word *gnosis* which is translated as 'knowledge' – not the kind of knowledge gained by rational study but a 'knowing' gained through a direct experience of God, including the practice of stilling the mind through meditation. I know little of these Gnostics, who have always been seen as heretics by the established church, but I come across their writings, once again, through a process of serendipity.

When my mother died, she passed down my father's extensive and eclectic library. At the time I had shelved his beloved books and always intended to take a closer look at some of the more esoteric works, but then life took over. Now, however, with time on my hands, I peruse the spines of his dusty tomes, and one title in particular seems to draw my eye – an English translation of the Gnostic 'Nag Hammadi' texts.

These texts, which were written sixteen hundred years ago, were found in 1945 by an Arab peasant combing a honeycomb of caves near the town of Nag Hammadi in Upper Egypt. There he discovered fifty-two scrolls of writing, which were subsequently examined by linguistic experts. Some of the texts were attributed (falsely, it is generally agreed) to Jesus' disciples, including *The Secret Book of James*, *The Apocalypse of Paul*, *The Apocalypse of Peter*, *The Gospel of Philip*, *The Letter of Peter to Philip*, and *The Gospel of Thomas*, the doubting wanderer who had travelled to India. These writings claim to record the secret sayings of Jesus which were said to contain hidden or secret knowledge known only by those closest to him, sayings that prioritize the importance of an individual and immediate experience of God over adherence to rational dogma.

It is thought these heretical Gnostic texts were initially hidden to prevent them being burned by the likes of Bishop Irenaeus of Lyon during the establishment of the 'catholic' and universal church. However, driven by my insatiable curiosity, I begin to read, and much of what I find in the pages of these Gnostic 'gospels' makes me deeply uncomfortable. I soon realize that there is much in Gnostic teaching that I profoundly reject, such as the dismissal of the idea of the bodily resurrection, the argument that the God of the New Testament is different from the deity of the Old, or the assumption that, while on the cross, Jesus rose above the suffering of physical death. (For over two thousand years Christians have found comfort in the knowledge that in Jesus we have a God who understands, and meets us, in our suffering.) But my interest is piqued to find that certain texts point towards that more intuitive relationship with God, which Griffiths says we in the West need to rediscover.

The Gnostics interpreted Jesus' encouragement 'Ask and it will be given to you; seek and you will find' (Matthew 7:7) as a mandate to seek their own personal experience of God. The non-canonical text *The Gospel of Thomas*, for example, claims to record Jesus saying that 'the kingdom is inside you and it is outside you. When you know yourselves, then you will be known, and you will understand that you are children of the living Father. But if you do not know yourselves, then you dwell in poverty, and you are poverty' (03:3–5).[1]

Some of the writings also refer to an experience of God that seems to be transcendent. One of the Gnostic authors writes of his own mystical experience, 'How shall I tell you about the universe? I am mind, and I see another mind, one that moves the soul . . . I have found the beginning of the power above all powers, without beginning' (58:31–61:2).[2]

The authenticity and the accuracy of the Gnostic texts (which weren't written until the second century) are questionable, but as I look even further back to sources that are regarded as canon, I also find references to mystical experiences. The apostle Paul, for example, claimed to have discovered 'secret wisdom, a wisdom that has been hidden and that God destined for our glory before time began' which he said that he shared only with Christians who were 'mature' (1 Corinthians 2:6–7). He wrote that he himself was 'caught up to the third heaven – whether in the body or out of the body I do not know' and there, in a trance, he heard 'things that cannot be told, which man may not utter' (2 Corinthians 12:2–4 ESV).

As I read and consider, I cannot help but wonder: *Is it too far-fetched to think that, in my moment of extremis, the poison of sepsis in my system had engendered a similar experience and that, as I sank beneath the waves of consciousness, I somehow tapped into this more intuitive connection with God?*

18

Kingdom Glimpses

Martin's decline comes very rapidly, although not without warning. Only a week previously, we had sat in my garden drinking tea; two bald-headed chemotherapy patients sheltering from the glorious spring sunshine under a large parasol. Once my hair had gone the way of all flesh it had been impossible to keep my condition from Martin and, as anticipated, he had not taken the news well. No matter how positive my own demeanour, he seemed to see the recurrence of my cancer as a portent of his own doom. Nevertheless, as we sat together on that beautiful spring day, he still seemed remarkably upbeat and resilient. However, in a private moment, his wife confided that he had refused to have the most recently offered scan out of fear that it might reveal further progression of the cancer. Instead, he preferred to pursue a policy of blissful ignorance.

To date, his ostrich-like approach had seemed to serve him rather well; he was still driving all over the countryside, planning an extension to their house, enjoying substantial meals and an evening whisky, and looking far better than I would have expected, given the advanced stage of his cancer.

So, even though the writing is on the wall, it still comes as a shock when I receive Cheryl's text saying that Martin has suffered a seizure and has been taken to hospital. My friend is in pieces, and my heart aches for her, but there's nothing I can do to help except pray and keep sending supporting messages (although I do activate the local prayer chain and ask them to pray for both my friends). Until, on the third day, the phone call comes.

Sadly, his passing had not been easy. His relentless denial of the seriousness of his situation meant that he had refused hospice care so, instead of being softly carried away on a cushion of morphine, he had not gone gently into that good night.[1] The following day would have been his birthday. My heart breaks for my friend.

Martin was not a churchgoing Christian, although I believe that he was on a journey and I hope that in his final hours he met his Maker. I can't imagine how it must feel to go through the challenge of cancer without the ability to bring your situation to God in prayer; to face the dark night of the soul without that solace. The reality, of course, is that anyone facing illness will sometimes feel alone, even if surrounded by supportive family and friends. No matter how sympathetic, or even empathetic, others are, it's impossible for them to share your experience (not that you would ever want them to). But one of the most extraordinary aspects of Christian belief is that, in Jesus, we have a God who knows pain. He has been through every type of suffering imaginable – betrayal, rejection, fear, despair, the agonies of the cross and even death – and, because of his mortal experiences, he is able to meet us in our suffering and accompany us on our own journey through the valley of the shadow of death.

Martin's death, however, leaves me with many questions. *If we are all God's beloved children then why is one person healed and not another? Why does one person live to see another day, and the other have to leave this earth too soon, leaving behind broken hearts?*

I think one of the most deeply damaging suggestions is that our survival relates to the depth of our faith. There *were* times when Jesus gave credit to his 'patients' for their individual faith, suggesting it was a contributing factor to their healing. For example, when a woman fought her way through the crowds to touch the cloak of the passing Messiah in the belief that it would cure her of menorrhagia, he told her: 'Daughter, your faith has healed you. Go in peace and be freed from your suffering' (Mark 5:34). However, there were also plenty of occasions when it doesn't seem to have been important whether the person being healed had faith or not. It is very unlikely, for example, that every one of the recipients of Jesus' twenty or more mass healing sessions was a devout and faith-filled follower and, when Jesus healed a paralysed man at the Pool of Bethesda, the apostle John records that the fortunate man had no idea who his saviour even was (John 5:1–15). Throughout the centuries there has also been a long line of the sickly faithful, from the apostle Paul who cried to God in vain to relieve him of the ailment he called the 'thorn in my flesh' (2 Corinthians 12:7), to John Wimber, who ran a pioneering healing ministry and himself succumbed to cancer and heart issues. So, I don't believe for a minute that lack of healing can be put down to lack of faith.

What I have come to understand, however, is that God's healing, or *rapha*, takes many forms. There are aspects of my previous physical healing from cancer that are hard to explain. As the early scans by the radiographer revealed, the healing actually began even before my first treatment and, by the end of six cycles of chemotherapy, the tumours had shrunk down so much that my oncologist told me in bewilderment, 'I don't know what to do with you now. There's no black-and-white guidance on what to do in a situation like yours, and given how amazingly you are doing I am anxious not to under-treat you . . . so I am recommending surgery.'

My surgeon was then able to remove most, but not all, of the cancer, and I subsequently was told that I would be given radiotherapy to try to give me quality of life for as long as possible. After being irradiated every day for three weeks, I went back to see the surgeon. As we entered his office, he didn't speak, but just looked at me long and hard before turning round the report on his desk and pointing to the bottom line of the letter which said: 'there is no evidence of cancer in her body.'

I am so profoundly grateful that, against all odds, I survived, but realize now that perhaps the most profound healing that I experienced was the inexplicable sense of peace that I was given. I was heartbroken at the thought that I might have to leave my family, but somehow was never afraid. I wasn't in denial – I actually put my affairs in order and there is even a funeral plan – but I somehow knew that I was going to be all right, even if this meant that I couldn't be with my family. I was somehow able to hold two realities in my mind at once – the possibility that I might have to leave this earth earlier than I had hoped and that of physical healing – and somehow these two were not in tension. And now as I look back on that first cancer journey, I realize that God's *rapha* is something bigger than, and may not always include, a cure; that perhaps his greatest healing is simply that 'peace of God, which transcends all understanding' (Philippians 4:7).

By the time of Martin's funeral, I'm back in hospital again. This time I have a problem with my Porta Cath line feeding into the large vein above my heart. My whole chest and neck area has turned bright red, my temperature is soaring, my stomach is distended and I have severe pain in my side. At the A&E department I recognize the nurse, who rapidly ushers me into a side room away from potential contaminants. An emergency doctor examines me and advises that it's likely I have a blood clot in the Porta Cath and the resulting distortion may be pushing on an artery near my stomach. If the blood clot moves, the situation could be life-threatening so, despite my lack of immunity, I am judged sufficiently at risk to be put in the 'high alert' bay next to the nurses' station in the acute emergency ward while I wait for a specialist linear CT scan.

From this vantage point I'm able to witness the frenetic activity of the ward. The acute emergency ward is the main feeder from the A&E department and it's in full swing twenty-four hours a day, seven days a week. By the time I'm admitted the lights have been dimmed, but seriously ill patients continue to be admitted throughout the night – many scared and confused. The air is filled with bewilderment and pain. One woman cries out every couple of minutes throughout the night.

Sleep is not really an option; it's rather like trying to take a nap in the middle of Piccadilly Circus during rush hour. The woman in the bed beside me is making inarticulate, confused animal sounds – guttural cries rising from the depths of her being. Her mouth lies open like a gaping wound and I cannot help wondering: *Is this how we all end?*

Around three o'clock in the morning the bed opposite is occupied by a very distressed woman who seems very bewildered as to her whereabouts and tries to fight off the nurses, who minister to her with the patience of Job. As soon as she is left alone, she wets the bed and, unable to comprehend how to use the call bell, starts to shout at the top of her voice, 'Help me, help me!' It is heartbreaking. I say a silent prayer that God will ease her troubled mind.

Utterly exhausted, I finally begin to doze lightly, only to be woken by someone shouting, 'Get him out of here! Get him out. He's not allowed in here. Help me. Get him away!' I lift my head up to meet the gaze of the woman opposite who is full of confused outrage. I realize that she thinks I am a man because of my bald head! I try to reassure her, telling her my name is Kate and that I really am a woman, but she has worked herself into such a state that she's incapable of hearing me, or comprehending. A nurse comes to her bedside and she too tries to explain that I am a woman, despite my bald pate, but it's no good. She shouts at me for the rest of the night until she is hoarse.

Just after four o'clock, an elderly woman is placed in the bed next to mine and, unable to sleep, I introduce myself. She tells me that twenty years ago she had suffered from non-Hodgkin lymphoma and had endured several rounds of chemotherapy and bone marrow operations. Her prognosis had not been good, but against all odds she recovered and had been cancer free ever since. However, at the beginning of the lockdown she had begun to cough up blood. She hadn't wanted to bother her GP in the midst of the pandemic and, a year later, when she finally accessed medical care, her worst fears were confirmed: she had a large tumour in her lung and around six months to live.

She shares her tragic story without a shred of self-pity, even punctuating her tale with occasional laughter, and tells me calmly, 'I'm not having no more chemo. There's no way I'm going through that again. It's brutal. Just want to go home and see my dog and my daughter. I'll be fine.' I'm so moved by her courage and fortitude. A doctor comes, draws the curtain and shares more bad news with her, his voice carrying beyond the gossamer-thin partition. All I can do is pray for her as I try not to listen to the conversation. I feel like an interloper, eavesdropping on such a personal moment in this poor woman's life, but then incongruous chuckling emanates from behind the curtain and, when the veil is drawn back, she is smiling serenely.

Opposite me, a nurse tries to clean the shouting woman, who is now rolling in her own filth. From behind the curtain, I hear her shriek 'What are you doing to my body? Leave me alone!' But the nurse replies with aching tenderness and kindness as she gently calms the storm, cleaning and caring for her protesting patient. I imagine that if I were to draw back the blue medical curtain, I would glimpse Christ standing there elbow deep in her muck – Jesus who so readily touched the untouchable. I'm truly in awe of the true compassion in this place. It is the compassion of Christ; not a distant sympathy delivered from some lofty height but mercy in all its messiness delivered through these wonderful people.

The context is challenging, to say the very least, but every person who is admitted to the ward is treated with the most extraordinary kindness and compassion. Every cry for help – no matter how often repeated – is responded to with almost preternatural patience by the staff, who appear at bedsides like ministering angels. Every interaction is respectful, considerate, even loving, as these amazing people care for, heal, feed, clean and comfort their – not always grateful – charges. From the staff nurses to domestic staff, healthcare assistants to ward housekeepers, porters to ward clerks – I never once see a glimmer of impatience or frustration even at the end of a gruelling twelve-hour shift. Instead, I'm struck by the extraordinary resilience, camaraderie and wonderful offbeat humour.

There is, however, great sadness when the staff speak about the impact of the pandemic. One healthcare assistant tells me that this ward was the 'ground zero' for the local Covid response. It was here that the first patients came, suffered and, in too many cases, died. She tells me that the ward had been a place of terrifying chaos: 'It were dead scary. When I went and got it, didn't want to come in here. Didn't want to add to the problems here.'

I ask, 'What did you do then?'

'Stayed at home, just me and ma dog. I got it real bad, though. Thought I was dying.'

I am horrified by the thought that this carer was without care.

She carries on: 'He saved ma life, ma dog. Stayed by ma feet all the time. I couldn't breathe an' he went all over the place. He climbed up on ma chest. Then I started throwing up, and ma legs weren't working. So me and ma dog slept on the floor outside the loo.'

It's an appalling tale told without self-pity, and I have to ask, 'How long were you off for?'

'Four months. Soon as I felt better, came back in. Was real scared still, but whad'ya do?'

I gaze at her in awe. Even after nearly dying from Covid, she just had to come back to this place – driven by a need to care for others that was too strong to ignore.

The realization hits me that there's no way I could have done this – I just don't have it within me – but that in these hospital wards I'm being granted a glimpse of God's kingdom: a diverse community of caring, selfless people, relentlessly putting others' needs before their own and doing so with kindness, compassion and even love. A community of people who, in our upside-down society, are some of the least recognized while corporate CEOs peddling fast food and superfluous consumer goods receive mind-boggling pay cheques and reality-show celebrities bask in undeserved recognition.

The journalist within me rails at the injustice. It seems so grossly unfair, but the Bible tells us that this is not God's ultimate plan for our world. As Jesus said, in God's kingdom 'the last will be first, and the first will be last' (Matthew 20:16). All those who have scrabbled so hard to secure the best seats at the top table will be asked to give them up to those who deserve them most in society. And when that day comes, it will be those who have cared, healed, fed, cleaned and comforted us when we needed them who will be seated alongside our Lord in the places of honour.

In the meantime, I know that Christ is somehow here in this place, in the healing hands and the patience, but also in the cries of pain and fear; unseen but all-pervading. I find I am seeing with new eyes, and in this place of suffering I am beginning to understand more fully that Christ, like the air, is all around us, and that in some indefinable way he is part of the reality I inhabit. That when I sank beneath the waves, he was the water that embraced me, 'for in him we live and move and have our being' (Acts 17:28). In his profound letter to the Ephesians, the apostle Paul explains that while we live out our lives in the seen world, we also dwell in an unseen heavenly or spiritual realm – a state which Paul calls being 'in Christ' and which Jesus described as 'abiding' in him. Our eyes may not see and our ears may not hear, but our spirit and soul affirms the presence of Christ permeating every atom of the known universe, and in this place I begin to grasp something of that mystery.

The pandemic has placed extreme pressure on the UK's healthcare system and, when Martin is laid to rest, I'm still waiting for my specialist CT scan and too unwell to leave the ward. My eldest comes down from Yorkshire to represent me at the funeral, but I am distressed at being unable to attend and heartbroken that I cannot be with Cheryl as she says a last goodbye to her husband of forty-plus years. I ask the nurse if it would be safe for me to make my way to the day room in order to spend some time in quiet reflection away from the chaos of the ward. She agrees on condition that I don't go 'running any marathons' and, taking my arms, helps me to walk unsteadily to a light bright room overlooking a courtyard of flowers. She sits me down in one of two armchairs beside a ward library shelf of Catherine Cooksons.

It seems an incongruous place to say goodbye but, at the time the service starts, I bow my head and say the Celtic blessing that I prayed at my aunt's funeral on Corfu:

Go on your journey from this world
carried by God who made you and loves you.
May the homeward path rise to meet you
and may you be welcomed across the threshold
and received in love's embrace.
For you, there is no more death or sorrow or pain.
So may the company of heaven enfold you
And keep you in peace this day and always.[2]

Then, as I sit in silence and sorrow, a realization comes to me. Martin didn't need to 'come to Christ' because Christ was already there with him, surrounding him every moment of his life. You can't come to that within which you already dwell. All you need to do is open the eyes of your heart to recognize this amazing reality – and, as Jesus told us, it is never too late for this to happen. In this life we may only see through a glass darkly, but as my daughter and Martin's loved ones watch his coffin disappear into the final flame accompanied by the strains of 'Wild Thing', I am certain that the veil has been drawn back and that my friend is now seeing the full glory of Christ face to face (1 Corinthians 13:12).

19

Limbo

The wait for a scan continues and, as the days roll by, the lack of sleep begins to take its toll. The full effects of the latest chemotherapy cycle also begin to make themselves felt and I shake constantly, my mouth so full of sores that it hurts to even drink water. Once again, I seem to be sinking fast and, ironically in this place of healing, I appear to be getting worse rather than better.

My husband emerges at my bedside each day after work armed with a bunch of bananas – one of the few things that I'm still able to eat. Tall, tanned and a vision of health, he looks so out of place sitting by my sickbed. At a loss as to how to deal with the situation, he fidgets and looks uncomfortable and I feel for him. As the days go by, the bananas on my table pile up to the point where I could open a fruit shop. The nurses find it amusing, but I realize that bringing fruit is his way of showing me how much he loves me. These precious bananas are his 'language of love'.

As the wait continues, I'm attended by an array of different doctors but there is little progress in terms of a firm diagnosis. I'm also visited on a regular basis by a phlebotomist who wryly refers to herself as 'the vampire'. I almost feel sorry for her as she struggles to find a vein, but howl like a baby as she digs around with a syringe in search of blood. The veins in my lymphoedema-free arm seem to have gone into permanent hiding, so options are limited.

On the day I was admitted, the nurse on duty had had a nightmare trying to get a cannula into the back of my right hand, which is now black and red and throbs with pain. My arm is on fire and I worry about an infection but am told to guard this cannula with my life as it's apparently the only way to get any fluids or treatment into my body. I'm trying hard to stay positive but feel stuck, waiting to find out the diagnosis for the fire and pain in my chest and belly, never mind treatment.

That night is particularly busy and by morning there are two new faces in my bay. As daylight creeps along the ward floor, the new cast of inmates check one another out. In the bed next to mine is a young woman who has screamed her way through the night but now seems calmer. She doesn't speak but turns and smiles at me feebly. I say a silent prayer for her. On the next bed, a woman of about 40 with closely cropped hair in leggings and a large baggy T-shirt sits hunched and grey-faced – she looks like a bewildered and frightened child. I go through the now familiar routine of asking her name and the reason for her admittance. Her answer saddens me – she has taken an overdose.

I clamber off my bed, weave my way unsteadily over to her and put out my hand. 'Should we?' she asks, but then puts her hand in mine and I hold it gently. In a trembling voice she tells me that she has had a row with her kids: 'It's too much . . .' She seems to hunch further into herself. 'They just say "Get on with it". I'm bipolar and they just don't get it.'

I explain that I grew up with someone who was bipolar and then just listen. For once, the rescuer in me doesn't try to provide any solutions; I just let her tell her story to someone who might just begin to understand. And as I listen to her struggles, some of which sound very familiar, I can't help but wonder whether God has brought the two of us together; whether there is some deeper rationale for why I am stuck waiting in this place.

That afternoon another of the beds in the bay is taken by a remarkably upbeat middle-aged woman with a large suitcase. She explains that she has a condition which brings her into A&E on a regular basis and usually keeps her in hospital for around ten to twelve weeks. She seems completely unfazed by her situation, is very well equipped for her stay, and greets all the nurses like old friends. Sitting cross-legged on her bed, she rummages in the bottom of her voluminous luggage and brings out a plastic bag full of tiny talismans – hundreds of tiny blue and silver guardian angels which she has crafted using tin and beads. I watch fascinated as she hands out these diminutive angels to any nurse, assistant or porter in the vicinity and each recipient beams with delight. It's as if this little gesture of gratitude lights a flame inside each of them and when they walk away their demeanour is transformed. When she comes to my bedside and hands me a blue and silver angel, I am moved by her kindness and clutch the divine messenger like my cross. Later on, when she walks over and also gives me a sleep eye-mask, I am almost speechless with gratitude – I could have kissed her.

That night the mask helps me to sleep for a while and I dream that a man in the hospital is selling time to impoverished and emaciated people whose time is running out. I stop a passing hospital porter and ask how much he has left, and he replies: 'Twenty minutes'. Hearing this, I'm enraged by the injustice and tell him, 'No you haven't. I'm going to stop the clock.' But before I can find out how I'm going to make time stand still, I'm dragged back into wakefulness. I have managed around three hours and, while welcome, it is not enough. I still feel ragged, worn down by lack of sleep and pain.

During the consultant's rounds, I ask again about when I might have the CT scan and I am told that a request has gone in but it is unlikely that there will be space for me today, or even tomorrow. Hearing this, something inside of me crumples and I start to cry and find I cannot stop. I fully give way to self-pity and am immediately appalled by its ugliness, but still can't stop the flood of tears.

> The waters have come up to my neck.
> I sink in the miry depths,
>> where there is no foothold.
> I have come out into the deep waters . . .
>> Psalm 69:1–2

A nurse comes to check my swollen bruised hand and points out that the cannula is too small to be used to inject the contrast dye necessary for the CT scan. So begins another half-hour of torture as she tries repeatedly to insert a larger cannula into the unwilling veins on the inside of my wrist, which only makes me cry harder. I feel like a 5-year-old.

My distress, however, does not go unnoticed and seems to prompt an escalation. I am visited by another doctor who, after conferring with the senior nurse, points out that I'm becoming progressively weaker and suggests that I might need to be moved to a quieter area. I'm also visited by the prayerful nurse who had been by my side through the Porta Cath insertion. She kneels beside my bed and, taking my hand in hers, kindly explains that the reason for the delay is that the CT scan has to be undertaken in an operating theatre in case I need to have immediate surgery, to remove either the clot or the Porta Cath – all of which will be undertaken under local anaesthetic. I'm grateful for the clarity but feel overwhelmed by the information and its implications – unsure whether I will be able to continue the lifesaving chemotherapy if the Porta Cath is removed – and I dissolve in tears yet again.

'I'm sorry I'm being so weak,' I sob into her shoulder.

'Even King David cried,' she tells me. 'The important thing is that we cry to the Lord.'

Then, in the middle of the busy ward, this extraordinary woman prays fierce and vocal prayers of healing over me. As she prays, my tears cease and, as I raise my head again, I beam into her beautiful face. I'm acutely conscious of the risk she runs in praying so openly on the ward but hope that those around me will be touched by her brave witness and God's healing. That night I sleep so soundly that in the morning the outgoing night-shift nurse tells me that I was snoring 'like a baby hippo'.

I'm barely awake when a message pops up on my phone from my prayerful friend telling me that I'm finally on the day's list of CT scans, and I'm still rubbing sleep from my eyes when she materializes at my bedside, together with a porter. She takes my hand and tells me, 'I wanted to come and be with you.' As the porter takes the brakes off my bed, she asks 'Where's your cross?' and, spotting it on the bedside table, grabs it for me as the bed is propelled out of the ward and down the corridor to the operating theatre.

I climb up onto the cold operating table and wince as the contrast dye runs in through the cannula in my swollen wrist and burns its way up my arm. I close my eyes and say a silent prayer. As I don't completely understand my condition, I am not really sure what to pray for, but remember that this really isn't important. So, as the scan proceeds, I plead to the Lord, 'Thy will be done.'

The scan is carried out by the radiologist who first inserted the Porta Cath and, after the interminable wait, the procedure is all over very quickly. I sense a slight defensiveness as he informs me that 'the Porta Cath is working perfectly well – it's in the right place', but he warms up as he delivers the good news that there is no blood clot in the line to my heart. I feel a squeeze of my hand and turn to my prayerful friend who is grinning from ear to ear. I say to the room in general, 'Thank you, Lord', adding my thanks to the radiologist, who says almost as an afterthought: 'There could be a blood clot in your arm, though. We will need to book you in for a further ultrasound scan.'

My heart sinks again as I wonder how long the waiting list will be for this scan. I seem to be stuck in an eternal limbo of waiting lists but, with some encouragement from my prayerful friend, the radiologist finally agrees to undertake the scan there and then. And again, to my huge relief, there are no blood clots; however, I still have no idea what *is* actually wrong with me!

On arrival back on the ward, I'm taken to a different area away from the main nurses' station. Now that the prospect of a life-threatening blood clot has been eradicated, I'm no longer regarded as critical and I am delighted to find myself in a larger, but much quieter, bay. That afternoon my sister

Charlotte breezes in, and as she arrives on the ward it's as if she is followed by the sun, which streams through an open window at the end of the bay. My sister has inherited my mother's relentlessly positive disposition and, while I am always determined to face the harsher realities of life head on, my sister always seems to see the best in every situation. Yet, despite our differences, the two of us share a deep bond forged by the experience of growing up within our loving and eccentric family. We had clung to each other through the deaths of our father, mother and later our aunt Theresa and, after their passing, we were drawn together by love and the knowledge that we were the last surviving members of our close-knit tribe. It was as if we spoke a language that only we two understood. As we talk, her natural optimism is infectious and, despite the pain, I begin to feel my spirits rising like sap.

Just before she leaves, I'm visited by the oncology team. The consultant explains that the blood work shows that I have an infection and to complicate matters my neutrophil count has once again plummeted to zero. My immune system is missing in action and, again, the threat of sepsis looms. The aim now is to get the infection under control and to prevent me from picking up any of the other bugs that inevitably swirl around a hospital and, in order to do this, I must once more be put in solitary confinement. Finally, the consultant tells me: 'If you keep on being this ill, we can't continue you on chemotherapy.'

I feel like a child who has been scolded. I'm angry at my body's inability to cope and am shaken by the prospect of the lifesaving chemotherapy being withheld. My sister does her best to comfort me but it's as if a cloud has passed over the sun. Before she leaves, she jokingly suggests that I'm going to have to adopt a 'monk-like' approach to this period in my life!

20

Solitude

That evening I'm moved to an isolation room, an IV of antibiotics is set up, the door closes and I am once again alone. The
sounds of the hospital are now distant and muffled, the quiet
wraps around me and I can hear myself breathe. The lack of
sound feels alien after the clamorous intensity of the acute
emergency ward.

As an extrovert I tend to be energized by the company of
others and my deepest fear has always been that of loneliness.
Since childhood I've nurtured a deep dread of involuntary
isolation – the bone-crushing loneliness of abandonment. But
something about this isolation is different. For some reason,
over the past few years, I have been increasingly fascinated by
the concept of spiritual retreat and the religious communities
where this discipline is most practised. Perhaps it's because the
members of these communities represent such a contrast to
my extroversion, focusing as they do on nurturing an introverted inner world of ideas and experiences.

While the collective church or the body of Christ is central
to the Christian faith, so is a more solitary and contemplative
relationship with God. It was Jesus himself who told his disciples, 'When you pray, go into your room, close the door and
pray to your Father' (Matthew 6:6), and he would also often

withdraw to come closer to his Father in prayer. The Gospel of Luke, for example, records that 'at daybreak, Jesus went out to a solitary place' (4:42). The Gospel of Mark also records God-incarnate encouraging his disciples, 'Come with me by yourselves to a quiet place and get some rest' (Mark 6:31), and this quiet place is sometimes translated as 'a desert place'. It's an interpretation which one group of early Christians known as the Desert Fathers took quite literally, leaving the madding crowds and heading out into the deserts of Egypt, Syria and Palestine in search of solitude, silence, and an experience of God that was specific and personal, rather than stereotypical or prescribed by others.[1]

Their withdrawal from society began around the beginning of the third century AD (about a hundred years before the Celtic Christians of the British Isles also began to see seclusion as central to a life of strict spiritual discipline) but picked up pace in the fourth century as the Roman emperor Constantine embraced Christianity and elevated it to a state religion. At this point the movement, which had been largely defined by exclusion and martyrdom, suddenly became mainstream and, while the number of those calling themselves 'Christians' burgeoned, some of the faithful felt confused. The faith of the earliest Christians had been sharpened and deepened by opposition, and some of the core faithful felt the need to once again separate themselves from the mainstream.

Their solution was to move away from the cities, where the new state-sponsored Christianity was becoming dominant, with a number of 'die-hards' retreating to the desert wilderness to find a different way of being a Christian in a rapidly changing world. Many of the 'Desert Fathers', as they became known, lived as hermits, and even those who lived in communities, such as the cenobites of Upper Egypt, kept their focus on solitude, stillness and silence. So the concept of monasticism was born (the terms 'monastic', 'monastery' and 'monk' deriving from the Latin word *monachos* which means 'single', or 'solitary').

The wisdom of these Desert Fathers was captured in a series of texts known as *The Sayings of the Desert Fathers* and in a series of interviews undertaken by the early Christian desert monk and theologian John Cassian (360–435). Cassian visited a number of monastic communities in the Egyptian desert of Scete and recorded his findings in two texts: the *Institutes* which outlines a model for monastic life that he applied in a monastery he founded in southern Gaul, near Marseille, and the *Conferences* which addresses the theology of the monks' spiritual and ascetic life.

The spiritual traditions and approaches recorded by Cassian went on to have a vast impact on the spirituality and practices of Western Christianity; Benedict of Nursia (480–548), for example, was hugely influenced by Cassian when he developed the Rule of St Benedict for monastic life, which in turn helped to shape medieval Europe. The influence of the Desert Fathers can also be seen in some medieval spiritual texts such as the anonymous fourteenth-century *The Cloud of Unknowing* which promoted a programme of silent prayer and meditation, and the *Spiritual Exercises* of Ignatius of Loyola (1491–1556) who founded the Jesuit movement.

I first ventured on my own spiritual retreat about ten years ago at Launde Abbey, an Elizabethan house and chapel set in rolling Leicestershire parkland. The house was built on the site of a twelfth-century Augustine priory which became a victim of Thomas Cromwell's dissolution of the monasteries.

In 1540 Cromwell wrote in his *Remembrances*, 'Myself for Launde', and hoped to build on the site and live there but, as he was executed for treason only three months later, it was his son George who first occupied the house that now stands there.

I stayed for three days in a simple upper room equipped with a single bed and desk, and slept beneath the watchful eye of the crucified Christ. During the days, I wandered in the footsteps of the Augustine monks, whose lives of quiet devotion modern visitors seek to emulate. Like the others who sought retreat at Launde, I spoke not a word during my time there. At first the concept of staying silent for days on end seemed alien to me. I had, after all, spent much of my life talking for a living – in churches, on the radio, on television and in the boardroom – and at first I felt compelled to fill the vacuum left by the departure of speech. But as I became accustomed to its absence, I realized that, far from being empty, the space left behind was pregnant with meaning. The silence itself seemed to have a voice that spoke without form to something deep within.

While working with World Vision, I went on to take some of my senior staff on retreat to the Benedictine Community of the Resurrection at Mirfield. Our planning meetings at the Community were punctuated by the hypnotic chanting of morning prayers, lunchtime Eucharist, evening prayer and Compline, the voice of one monk after another building layers of praise until the sound reverberated around the stone walls. At mealtimes we ate in the large refectory, seated together with the monks on long bench tables. Together we shared silent meals with our voiceless hosts and, after Compline, I walked in the gardens wrapped in silence before retiring to sleep.

Later, after leaving World Vision and beginning my career as an author, I also became a frequent visitor to a nearby Society of the Sacred Mission priory. The priory, which has since closed down, was only 10 miles from my home but I would often rent a room where I could spend time in solitude, praying and writing. Perhaps I was drawn to this more introverted world simply because writing is such a solitary pursuit; but, whenever I faced writers' block, when my mind churned like a storm-swept sea and I struggled to creatively frame my thoughts, I would return to the priory and, in the silence, I found I could see as clearly as if looking down into a still clear pool of water.

After a while the brothers took me under their wing; they gave me a space in their theological library to reflect and write, and gradually I was drawn by their gentle friendship deeper into the life of the priory. Once a week, I would arrive early and join the brothers for morning prayers before retreating to my garret room in the library to work. At midday we would silently process to the chapel for Communion, after which I joined the residents for a simple meal. Side by side, we would eat without commentary but in deep companionship.

I found something of great beauty and inestimable worth in the separation from sound and, although I would never be more than a visitor, I found it a great blessing to spend time alongside those who have the self-discipline to live a life so focused on God and are able to communicate so clearly their joy in the Lord without words; who recognize that God speaks in the silence. After all, when God spoke to Elijah it was not in the storm or the earthquake but in the quiet. And perhaps when we encounter the divine the most natural response is one of awe and reverential silence.

My current retreat in this isolation room is not voluntary like those of the past but, rather than feeling lonely, I find myself wrapped once again in a comforting blanket of silence and solitude. On reflection I realize that my room bears some resemblance to a retreat room or monastic cell; a place of solitude where, like the psalmist, I can wait alone in silence for God (Psalm 62:5). I decide that I will take my sister's advice and adopt a 'monk-like' approach to the situation, and begin by going back to one of the disciplines that I learned at the priory.

The roots of the monastic practice of *Lectio Divina* or 'divine reading' go all the way back to the third century, and it plays a central role within the Benedictine Rule. The practice involves repeatedly reading a piece of Scripture and dwelling within it in different ways; it's not about exegesis or interpretation of the text but rather a deep contemplation and meditation on the divine word. To read in this way you don't need to know the historical context or to understand the doctrinal implications of a text; rather it's about recognizing the Bible as the living word of God, the meaning of which is revealed to us by the Holy Spirit, and for many the discipline is seen as a gateway into a deeper relationship with God.

Lectio Divina involves four steps. First of all, *lectio*, the slow, gradual reading of a piece of Scripture, savouring every word and allowing them to settle within you. The second step is *meditatio*, or meditation on words or passages that seem to speak directly to you, allowing them to wash over you until the meaning begins to rise to the surface. Third, *oratio*, praying to God about what has been revealed and listening for what he may have to say specifically to you. And finally, *contemplatio*, a deep and silent dwelling with the word in the presence of God and a wordless expression of our love for him.

Revisiting this practice, I sit in the stillness of the afternoon sun and pick up my phone. I already subscribe to a number of daily devotionals and now open up the first one in my inbox which features a passage from the book of Jonah. And, as I slowly digest the passages, a sense of awe is born within me:

You hurled me into the depths,
  into the very heart of the seas,
  and the currents swirled about me;
all your waves and breakers
  swept over me.
I said, 'I have been banished
  from your sight;
yet I will look again
  towards your holy temple.'
The engulfing waters threatened me,
  the deep surrounded me;
  seaweed was wrapped around my head.
To the roots of the mountains I sank down;
  the earth beneath barred me in for ever.
But you, LORD my God,
  brought my life up from the pit.

When my life was ebbing away,
  I remembered you, LORD,
and my prayer rose to you,
  to your holy temple.

Jonah 2:3–7 NIV 2011

As I dwell with the words, I am taken back to the last time that I struggled in an isolation room: to that sense of surrender and the vivid experience of descending to the depths and the peace of the ocean floor – that liminal place where, enveloped in silence, I sensed something powerful and tangible. I sit in wonder, contemplating the words of this ancient mariner, and feel again that yearning to return to the ocean depths, to the shadowed wilds of the seabed of my mind, where I sensed the presence of the God who cannot be contained with words.

Unable to participate in the collective life of the church, I have been seeking to keep the embers of my faith alive by clinging to a self-imposed 'rule of life' – struggling to continue with my practice of reading the Bible, saying the Daily Offices and spending time in personal prayer even when I was so ill that I found it hard to read. As I have grown weaker, I have seen such disciplines as a way to impose a sense of structure on my life. But now I wonder whether they are in fact something much deeper. *Are these disciplines actually a gateway back to the depths and to that profound intuitive connection with God?*

21

New Rhythm

After four days of reflection and prayer, I am finally deemed sufficiently recovered to return home to the bosom of my family. My period of monastic retreat comes to an end and, as we head further into summer, I seem to enter a different phase of my journey.

On my next visit to the cancer centre, I am to start a new medical regime made up of a different form of chemotherapy called docetaxel and two monoclonal antibody treatments, trastuzumab and pertuzumab – extraordinary drugs that are specifically designed to treat HER2 cancer and work by locking on to the HER2 proteins on or in any cancer cells in your body. (Until the late 1990s, a diagnosis of HER2 cancer carried dire implications, but these amazing drugs provide new hope for patients like me.)

I'm already familiar with docetaxel, having been treated with this chemotherapy drug seven years ago, and after an initial infection I previously managed to tolerate the drug relatively well. So I'm now hopeful that I can get through the remaining chemotherapy cycles without any more trips to A&E. What is less certain, however, is how my body might react to the monoclonal antibody treatments. These wonder drugs come with many of the same side effects as chemotherapy, including lowered resistance to infection, tiredness, loss of appetite, and sickness, while trastuzumab carries additional risks for the heart, including irregular heartbeats or palpitations, damage to the muscle, and build-up of fluid around the heart. These are usually temporary but have to be monitored very carefully with regular echocardiograms.

So, ahead of the first round of the new treatment, I once again lay myself down on a narrow hospital trolley, the cold plastic clinging to the skin of my back as a radiologist presses a scanner into my chest. All I can hear is the sound of my heart, the rhythmic thudding of the engine of my body pumping life through my veins – a tempo that reminds me of those early sonograms when I was able to listen to my children while they were still in the womb. Mercifully, the echocardiogram shows that my heart should be strong enough to withstand the storm that is about to break, which I take as a sign that things are looking up.

I also meet my oncologist, who tells me he is delighted to say that my CT scan shows a significant reduction in the size of all three of the tumours. I almost hug him but instead, once I'm outside, I sit in the car park, pouring out prayers of gratitude. It now seems that all the complications of the chemotherapy over the past few months have been worth it and, when I go back to the cancer centre for my next round of treatment, I feel a renewed sense of purpose.

In order to ascertain which, if any, of the drugs a patient reacts to, the first round of the new treatments is divided up and given over a couple of days. I go for my first treatment on St Irenaeus's Day at the end of June and, as the first dose of trastuzumab flows into my veins, I meditate on the saint's famous words, 'The glory of God is a human being fully alive' – ancient wisdom and modern medicine. Mercifully there is no drastic reaction to the new treatment, apart from the usual steroid-induced insomnia, so I return the following day for the second targeted treatment, pertuzumab, which is once again administered without incident.

The plan is to give the new chemotherapy treatment, docetaxel, the same day but, due to my problems with the former type of chemotherapy, my oncologist has decreed that I should only be given 80 per cent of the potential dosage of this new drug. As I'm being hooked up to the IV, I feel prompted to ask the nurse, almost as an afterthought, 'This is an eighty per cent dosage, isn't it?' The question elicits an alarmed response. I'm about to be given a 100 per cent dose of docetaxel, which, I suspect, would have landed me back in hospital in a few days' time. I say a silent prayer of thanks that the error was spotted. It means that I will have to return for a third day to be given the correct dose, but I have probably been saved another trip to A&E.

The following day, the correct dose is finally administered and, as I emerge from the cancer centre, Maria, who is waiting patiently, says: 'You look like a different woman this time.' Apparently, every time I had emerged after previous treatments, I had seemed frail and bowed down, but this time she observes: 'You actually seem to have a spring in your step' – and as the days progress, a new rhythm of life begins to emerge.

For the first week after chemotherapy, I still spend much of my time drifting in and out of sleep but, when I finally resurface, I find that my health hasn't deteriorated as dramatically as previously. I still have fatigue, sickness, bleeding gums and searing pain when I eat, but it's now more bearable and after the seven days I begin to feel almost human again. The sap is rising within me and, by the final week of the cycle, my energy levels are so improved that I feel strong enough to venture out of the house.

Initially I only totter a couple of hundred yards down the short lane below our house, lean on the cross-bar gate and look out over the ripening crops which undulate light as they wave with the breeze. But as my strength returns I become more ambitious and day by day make my way further up the lane towards Cowper's Alcove. As my stride gradually lengthens I fall into a rhythm, and my steps, like those of the early Celtic saints, are accompanied by the inward poetry of the Psalms:

> When I consider your heavens,
>   the work of your fingers,
>   the moon and the stars,
>   which you have set in place,
>   what is man that you are mindful of him . . .?

                                                              Psalm 8:3

Having committed the beauty of these words to heart, I now carry them within me like precious jewels and, as I walk in the early cool of the day, they rise up within me and fall like morning dew. Eventually, as I attain the summit crowned by Cowper's Alcove, I bathe in the captured sunlight and gaze over the ancient landscape. My heart races – an unexpected joy rises in my heart. I'm struck by profound gratitude that I am here on this planet today, looking up into the clear blue sky, and begin to feel a sense of anticipation. When my sister drives up from London, she is amazed to find me sitting happily in the garden, my grin protected by a large sunhat. When she posts a picture of me on Instagram, she adds a comment that I seem to be made of steel girders. Steel, however, doesn't bounce and I prefer to think that God has injected some rubber into my soul! I am beginning to heal in more ways than one.

Until now I have been daunted by the side effects of the treatment but, as I go for my next chemotherapy cycle, I find that I am now able to willingly surrender and even embrace the process, because I know that it is in the aftermath of treatment that I seem to come closest to another tantalizing glimpse of my 'ocean floor' experience of God. The chemical clouding of my mind actually seems to help me towards a more intuitive perception; it seems that it's only when I give up the struggle to think clearly that my mind is set free to roam to the depths of my consciousness in search of him. As time goes on, I also become more confident that I will rise again to the surface, clutching to my heart whatever treasures he has revealed to me, and, as my energy gradually returns after each chemotherapy cycle, I am left with nostalgia and yearning for that almost transcendent sense of closeness that I once found in the depths.

I still begin the day listening to God's word, joining other Anglicans in reciting the morning liturgy, and spending time in personal prayer as well as an increasingly voluminous intercession for the many I know who are suffering in body, mind and spirit. But I still feel as if I am skating over the surface of a deeper reality. Despite the profundity and beauty of the words of the Bible and the liturgy, I recognize that they are nevertheless only signposts to the divine mystery that cannot be contained by language – the God whose thoughts are so far beyond our thoughts that our imagination cannot do him justice. It's as if I am treading in the shallows while what I yearn for is to connect with the ineffability of God that lies beyond the safety of the shore and white-capped waves – to relive that experience granted to me in my hour of greatest need as I lay on the ocean floor. So, like countless others over the centuries, I close my eyes and seek, within the stillness, the awesome presence of God.

22

Exploration

There's a common theme that ties together the spiritual lives of the early Christians – including the apostle Paul, the Desert Fathers, the Celtic saints, the medieval monastics such as St Benedict and the twentieth-century spiritual master Bede Griffiths – and that is the drive to seek a more intuitive experience of God through meditation.

In his wonderful biography of the apostle Paul, Tom Wright talks about a practice of prayer and meditation which goes all the way back to Abraham and was embraced by the Jewish sages of the first century AD. These early practitioners would focus on a passage of Scripture with the hope of gaining a mysterious *apokalypsis*, or revelation, of the ultimate mystery of heaven. According to Wright, one of the central texts associated with this meditation is the opening chapter in the book of Ezekiel with its psychedelic descriptions of the throne of heaven, a flashing wheeled chariot and four-faced angels, and he suggests that Paul, a devout Pharisee, might have been engaged in such a meditation on the journey to Damascus, and envisages the journey unfolding:

In his mind's eye, then, he has the four-faced creatures and the wheels. He focuses on them. He sees them. He ponders them.

Will he dare to go further? Upward, with prayer and quickening pulse, to the chariot itself. Was it his imagination? Was he actually seeing it? Were his eyes open, or was it just his heart's eyes opened to realities normally invisible? . . . Upward again, then, to the lower part of what seems to be a figure on the throne, some kind of human form . . . He is seeing now, eyes wide open, conscious of being wide awake but conscious also that there seems to be a rift in reality, a fissure in the fabric of the cosmos, and that his waking eyes are seeing things so dangerous that if he were not so prepared, so purified, so carefully devout, he would never have dared to come this far. Upward again, from the chest to the face. He raises his eyes to the one he has worshipped and served all his life . . . And he comes face-to-face with Jesus of Nazareth.[1]

This theory is supported by Paul's own account in his second letter to the Corinthians of a transcendent, spiritual encounter in which he says he was 'caught up in the third heaven'. There he encountered Christ and heard 'things that cannot be told', a wisdom hidden to others (2 Corinthians 12:2–4 ESV). (It was this 'secret wisdom' (1 Corinthians 2:7) that the Gnostics also claimed to seek through spiritual practices such as meditation.)

The Desert Fathers also practised a form of meditation which was referred to as *quies* or *hesychasm* (after *hesychia*, the Greek for quiet and stillness). Their aim was to achieve inner silence, emptying their minds of all thoughts and images, aided by the repetition of a short phrase – in particular the Jesus Prayer: 'Lord Jesus Christ, Son of God, have mercy on me, a sinner' (which in shortened form became the Kyrie Eleison: 'Lord, have mercy'). This in turn influenced the development of the Benedictine *Lectio Divina* and some of the mystic meditative practices of medieval Europe.

The Cloud of Unknowing, an influential spiritual work by an anonymous fourteenth-century author, also states that God lies beyond the reach of human intellect and that the only way we can pierce the 'cloud of unknowing' that lies between us and God is by abandoning all thoughts in meditation and silent prayer. This is the 'work' of contemplation, which in medieval times referred to seeking a soul's union with God.[2] Until the Middle Ages, it was thought that only those who had chosen monastic life could engage in such meditative contemplation, but by the fourteenth century it had become accepted that even those who had outwardly active lives were capable of seeking God in the silent cloud of unknowing. In fact, works like *The Cloud* kick-started the popularization of meditative techniques. Now I, too, am drawn towards this approach that involves laying aside my habitual rationalism in order to reach beyond 'knowing' and thought in the hope of 'union with God'.

In some respects, the mysticism of the Byzantine meditative techniques are not that far removed from the eastern tradition that so influenced Bede Griffiths during his time in India. The meditation method that was taught by Griffiths is a form of Christian meditation that draws on Hinduism and Buddhism. However, the aim of Hindu and Buddhist meditation differs from that of the Christian, which seeks that point of our own being where we encounter the Holy Spirit of God.

The Christian meditation taught by Bede starts with a seated *asana* position that prepares the mind to be still through the relaxation of the body. Having reached postural stillness, he recommends stilling the mind through a focus on the breath as it moves in and out of the body. This is followed by the repetition of the Jesus Prayer, 'Lord Jesus Christ, have mercy on me, a sinner', until the mind eventually becomes still and we find that 'inner reality that is open to the transcendent'.[3]

Some of what Griffiths writes resonates with my own experience, although my feelings about meditation to date have been rather mixed and bear little connection to my Christian faith. For instance, I first encountered the practice at university, where I had a brief flirtation with Transcendental Meditation. TM is a form of silent meditation that was developed in the fifties by the Indian guru Maharishi Mahesh Yogi, and was popularised in the 1960s by The Beatles.

In the 1980s a fellow student, who I had a bit of a crush on, invited me to attend a weekend TM retreat in a woodland centre in the foothills of the Cambrian mountains. I was still in my 'anger-with-God phase' so was resistant to trying anything that smacked of religion but, despite its Vedic roots, TM was sold as a non-spiritual discipline aimed at personal well-being, its benefits ranging from 'inner peace' to lowering blood pressure.

The local Welsh 'guru' gave us each a single word or phrase, a 'mantra', like those used by the Desert Fathers, which was presented to us individually by our teacher (I'm ashamed to say I can't actually remember what mine was), and we sat in a circle of chairs in the garden, lost in our own inner realities. Initially my attempts at inner peace were hampered by my own internal noise which seemed to intensify the more I tried to clear my mind. Eventually, however, the incessant inner chatter began to quieten and, as my thoughts parted, I found myself gazing inwardly into a dark space where slowly but surely visual impressions began to emerge. At first, they were abstract and amorphous, drifting across my inner vision like the pulsating blobs in a lava lamp. But gradually I noticed a pulsating pinprick of light which eventually seemed to explode and expanded into a horizontal field reaching endlessly in every direction, opening up the darkness to infinity. It was an extraordinary experience in an unashamedly secular retreat, and while I doubt it had any deep spiritual significance, it piqued my curiosity about the nature of consciousness and my inner reality.

During my travels in Asia I also attended a couple of Theravada Buddhist meditation classes in Thailand and then experimented with Mahayana Buddhist meditation while in Dharamsala in northern India. I limited my experimentation to *samatha* meditation which involves mindfulness of the breath. *Samatha* is one of the most ancient but also the simplest and most recognizable forms of meditation. Once you are settled into a comfortable meditation position, you close your eyes and focus your mind on the rising and falling of the breath as it passes in and out of the body, and as thoughts begin to distract your attention you simply let them pass like clouds in the sky, bringing your awareness back to the breath flowing in and out of your body. The word *samatha*, which comes from the Pali language, means 'calm'.

I was not a good student, however, and after only the briefest of studies, I turned away from Buddhism – and associated meditative practice – as I found myself unable to comprehend a reality that didn't include God. In fact, if anything, my brief foray into Buddhist meditation only served to drive me further along on my journey back towards Christ. Now, however, as I recall my early experiences with meditation, I remember being told that our mental state can be compared to an ocean, our thoughts being like the waves on the surface of the sea, and that the aim of the meditation is to reach down to the transcendent stillness in the depths.

So, I begin to explore, starting with Christian mindfulness. Secular mindfulness has become something of a trend over the past few years. Developed by Jon Kabat-Zinn in the 1970s, it is seen as a means of becoming aware of, and recognizing our independence from, negative thought patterns – enabling the realization that we are not our thoughts. While the concept undoubtedly springs from centuries of religious practice in Asia, it has now been denuded of any religious content or connotations and is focused purely on achieving a state of alert relaxation by paying attention to the present moment, our thoughts, and our bodily sensations including our breath. For some it provides a valuable retreat from the busyness of life and, for others, a means of overcoming the darkness of our own thoughts. But in recent years there have been leaders who have also looked at the practice from a Christian perspective, viewing mindfulness as something different – a means of tapping into our innate capacity for awareness of God; a capacity that seems to be hardwired into our very nature but which atrophies with exposure to the pressures of the world. As such, Christian mindfulness is about obeying the biblical prompting to stop the endless cycle of human activity – even those tasks carried out in the service of God – and allowing ourselves to simply 'be' and know that he is God. It's about following Jesus' example, spending time alone in prayer, obeying the Sabbath command to set aside a time which is holy – when we rest from our labours and concentrate on simply being in his presence.

As a very action-oriented personality type, I've always found simply 'being' rather than 'doing' quite challenging. In the Gospel of Luke there's a wonderful description of two sisters, Martha and Mary, who were friends of Jesus. Luke describes how, when Jesus visited them, Martha welcomed him in and then busied herself with preparations that needed to be made for his stay. While Martha scurried around, her sister Mary went to sit at Jesus' feet, listening to what he had to say, until finally the harassed sister cracked and accosted Jesus, saying: 'Lord, don't you care that my sister has left me to do the work by myself? Tell her to help me!' To which Jesus replied, 'You are worried and upset about many things, but only one thing is needed. Mary has chosen what is better, and it will not be taken away from her' (Luke 10:40–42).

For most of my life I've definitely been a bit of a 'Martha', always busy with tasks – both secular and spiritual. But what God now seems to be showing me through this cancer experience is that the time has come to be more like Mary; to learn how to simply *be* in the moment, taking time to simply exist. It's also not lost on me that the profound 'ocean floor' experience that I had of him came at a time when I was forced to be still as a result of my illness, and I suspect that, if I am once again obedient to the call to stillness, I will perceive him more clearly. Ultimately, I must finally learn to be mindful, not in the secular sense of the word, but the spiritual.

There are quite a number of resources available to Christians who want to explore mindfulness from a faith perspective, ranging from apps to online courses, but I choose the teaching of a soft-spoken Scotsman called Richard H.H. Johnston. The author of several books on mindfulness, Johnston is one of the founding leaders of the UK National Mindfulness Day for

Christians and the Mindful Church. I heard Johnston speak at a conference a few years ago about how, by detaching yourself from negative thought patterns, you can create a space where you can experience and rest in the love, grace and kindness of God. Now I am particularly struck by his argument that mindfulness helps with the process of surrendering to God through acceptance of the moment and all that it brings. As Johnston points out, 'the present moment may not always be a pleasant one',[4] but in order to be truly mindful of the presence of God you need to surrender your sense of control; to be willing to fully inhabit the moment, no matter how painful, and to walk through the waters rather than avoiding or circumnavigating them. So, one Monday morning, after the front door closes and silence descends, I begin learning the skill of mindfulness.

At the core of this practice lies the breath – the focal point of many types of meditation and secular mindfulness. But in Christian meditation the breath takes on new resonance as it's seen as symbolic of life itself: the animation given to us by God when he breathed our dust-formed selves into existence. The Hebrew word used for that breath in the account of Adam's genesis is *ruach*, which also means 'Spirit'. God breathed his very Spirit into humanity, and while breath continues there is life. The act of breathing is one of those essential bodily functions that really does operate on autopilot. In general, most of us will breathe around 23,000 times a day, and if we live to the age of 80 we will have taken more than 672,760,000 breaths – most of which will have passed completely unnoticed. But the reality is that each breath is a God-given miracle sustaining our existence, and it is the cessation of breath that tells others when our life here on earth has come to an end.

So now I turn my attention to this miraculous breath and, as I close my eyes, settle my limbs and mind, and turn my focus inwards, I recognize how blessed I am to still be breathing. As I focus on the rising and falling of my abdomen, I'm filled with an overwhelming gratitude for the breath in my lungs, and slowly I feel my body begin to relax like a coil unwinding and my mind begins to settle. My breath flows in and out like the ebb and flow of the tide and, lulled by the natural rhythm, I enter my interior world, where I sit and wait in anticipation.

In meditation, the idea is to go into the process without expectation; to let go of any kind of goal setting, no matter how spiritual, and to be content with whatever the process brings. But I find it hard to let go of the desire to once again plumb the depths, to turn off the anticipation of that profound connection, and, noting this yearning, I have the sense that I am somehow *not doing this right*. Thoughts begin to intrude. I try to shut off the judgmental voice inside my head and to view emerging thoughts as clouds drifting across the inner clear-blue expanse, rather than following them down a rabbit hole of reasoning. But my mind continues to probe, providing an accompanying narrative to the process of meditation.

At first, I find it almost impossible to let go of each thought but, as the days go by, I begin to relax into the process until my thoughts drift – one by one – across my mind and eventually pass out of view, leaving behind a clear blue sky. Occasionally the thoughts that pass before my mind's eye seem to have come from God, glimpses of profundity that I want to explore further. The writer within wants to capture each insight, knowing that once they drift out of view of my chemo-addled brain they will be gone for good. But mindfulness teaches us to let go of even these thoughts, so reluctantly I let them pass.

Eventually my focus expands to my whole body and it's as if my whole being is breathing in and out, pulsing with each breath. As I breathe, I feel my soul expanding, opening and reaching out, until I am flooded with a sense of well-being, peace and calm that I know can only come from him, my Jehovah Rapha. I sit resting in the moment, awake but with no desire to turn to wakefulness, until the toll of a bell brings me back into the day.

To my delight, the next lesson involves chocolate. Since my first cancer diagnosis I've severely limited my intake of sugar and, over the past seven years, chocolate has been a very rare treat – restricted to celebrations such as Easter, Christmas and birthdays. But now, in the cause of spiritual development, I've been given permission to crack open a bar, the idea being to connect with the world through our God-given senses.

In slow motion I unwrap the bar, taking in every detail, from the artificial smoothness of the plastic wrapper to the powdery ridges scoring the surface of the chocolate. Breaking off a square, I close my eyes and first bathe in the sweet's heady floral aroma before placing it on my tongue. I resist the urge to chew but rather allow it to sit in my mouth, gradually melting into my taste buds, until a sumptuous earthy stream of chocolate runs down my throat. I can't remember ever having tasted anything so utterly delicious and exotic. It feels like such a guilty pleasure, but I get the point that in order to experience God we have to experience life in all its multifaceted wonder. Unlike those who take up the contemplative life, we, who live out in the world, spend so much of our time on autopilot, unaware of the sanctity of any given moment. Brother Lawrence (a lay brother who served as a cook for the severe order of Discalced Carmelites in Paris in the seventeenth century), for example, believed that every moment and every action, no matter how mundane, presents an opportunity to practise the presence of God, and perhaps that extends to the simple sensual pleasure of eating chocolate. There are still puritan undercurrents in some Christian circles that lead us to believe that such pleasures are a sin, and I've lost count of how many times I've given up chocolate for Lent. But the point being made is that all of our senses – including that of taste – were part of God's plan when he created us. Which is why the practice of Christian mindfulness taps into these senses as a way of becoming more aware of the presence of God.

In his book *Introducing Christian Mindfulness*, Johnston points to the integration of body, soul and spirit as expounded by the apostle Paul in 1 Thessalonians 5:23, and recommends this form of meditation as a way of encouraging 'the development of mindful awareness in all areas of the integrated self'.[5] He also argues that an over-spiritualized denial of the flesh runs counter to the biblical teaching that 'your body is a temple of the Holy Spirit, who is in you, whom you have received from God' (1 Corinthians 6:19–20). Right now, my body feels more like a cracked vessel than a temple, but everything I have experienced leads me to believe that there is treasure within. If connecting with my body – including its pain – will enable me to better understand and connect once again with God at a deeper level, then I feel that this is something I must persevere with.

I lie on my bed listening to a bird singing in the tree outside, then close my eyes and deepen each breath. Slowly, I become aware of the pressure points where my back and legs press into the mattress, and my skin tingles with the gentle caress of the breeze coming through the open window. I begin to relax and simply enjoy lying here.

Following the instructions of my digital tutor, I continue with a Mind and Body meditation by focusing attention on my right foot, breathing into my body right down to my toes, and am surprised by sensations that no doubt continually exist but which I am actually noticing for the first time. Then, slowly but surely, I work my way up my body, the focus moving to my ankle, then to my calf, knee and thigh. I repeat the exercise with my left leg, then work my way up through my torso, arm and neck to my face.

As I focus my attention on different parts, I become acutely aware of nerve endings firing all over my anatomy – and of my brokenness. Every part of my body groans, the chemotherapy having burnt its way into my being. The pain courses through my old surgery scars and into my right side as the chemotherapy attacks the tumours like a chemical Pacman. My mouth and throat burn, the rawness standing out in sharp relief. I realize that on a daily basis I have been waging a war of mind over matter, trying to block out all the signals that my ailing body has been sending me.

Now I am electrically aware of every fibre of my cancer-invaded body and, as I lie with this knowledge, there is a creeping acceptance that I am what I am: a broken jar of clay, whose pieces are still loved. As my mechanisms of denial break down and the pain floods my body, I lie with the awareness of my brokenness and feel a sense of overwhelming gratitude. I feel so utterly alive, vibrant and aware. It wouldn't matter if I could never move again, because I feel that I am completely loved, and I thank the Lord for the great gift of my body with all its imperfections.

As I continue with the course, I also discover a practice called Mindfulness of Movement, an idea that resonates with my experience of finding peace when travelling. My horizons are now limited, but one morning, when I feel well enough, I try to walk 'mindfully' up the lane towards Cowper's Alcove – my precious prayer space. I focus my awareness on every muscle, the effortless swinging of an arm, the stretch of a calf as I step forward and the pressure of my shoes as they beat the earth beneath my feet. As I walk, a horse approaches, the syncopation of its hooves on the ground vibrating through my body and, once the rider has passed, the rhythmic pattern of the hooves gradually fades away like the sound of a Tibetan singing bowl, until I am once again alone.

A large striped bumble bee proceeds languorously ahead of me up the lane and, out of the corner of my eye, I spot a small muntjac deer as it runs across the newly ploughed field, graceful, free and majestic. A brimstone butterfly rises up before me, resplendent, cloaked in pale-yellow glory, followed by seemingly random thoughts: *Why did God make the universe in colour? It's such an extravagant gesture – he could have easily made the world in black and white. And does God perceive colour the same way that we do (dogs see colour differently, so why not God)?* It is a few minutes before I realize that I am once again galloping after a train of thought, and bring my focus back to the rhythmic movement of my body through the summer morning.

Like my Celtic Christian ancestors, I am lost in wordless praise at the beauty of the world around me, the earth beneath my feet – the stuff from which I was made, and the boundless expanse of the sky above with its intimation of eternity. I simply savour the cool breeze on my face, invisible and intangible, passing in and out of my lungs. I know that in a few days the next round of chemotherapy will render me once again inert, but for now I stride out, revelling in the moment, arms slicing through the air that seems electric with his presence: *In him I live and move and have my being, Christ before me, Christ behind me, Christ beneath me, Christ above me, Christ on my right, Christ on my left and Christ within me.*

23

Shoreline

One day I receive an email from my rector informing me that, after almost two years of Covid restrictions, he is finally able to administer Holy Communion at home. I am thrilled and grasp the opportunity with both hands. One of my greatest privations has been not being able to participate in the sacrament of the Eucharist. My own church had made the decision not to stream their services online, so for over a year I had faithfully logged on to the diocesan online services from my tiny home office, and tried to will myself into the heart of the experience as I watched the bishop or archdeacon consuming bread and wine – hoping to share spiritually, if not physically, in this ancient rite. But eventually, even these online services came to an end and, cut loose, I roamed the internet sampling some of the less traditional offerings from the likes of Holy Trinity Brompton and the Soul Survivor Church in Watford. I entered into the experience – singing along enthusiastically, if not tunefully, with various worship bands – which I found uplifting. But I was still left with a feeling that something was missing.

There's something profound about the rhythm of a eucharistic service; the way it gathers us into God's house to confess our failings, praise him, and then invites us to the Lord's Table to re-enact that pivotal moment in the life of Christ and humankind. That Passover night when, knowing that he was betrayed by the sin of humanity, God-incarnate broke bread and shared it with his disciples, saying: 'Take and eat; this is my body', and lifting one of the four ritual cups of Passover wine gave thanks and offered it to his disciples, saying: 'Drink from it, all of you. This is my blood of the covenant, which is poured out for many for the forgiveness of sins' (Matthew 26:26–28).

I still have vivid memories of how I felt the first time I was asked to assist in the Communion service at our church. As I stood beside the rector at the altar, it was if I had entered a place of mystery where I stood on the border between the natural and the supernatural, the seen and unseen. As I watched the rector lift up the ordinary things of this earth, praying 'grant that by the power of your Holy Spirit these gifts of bread and wine may be to us his body and his blood',[1] and as I stepped forward and placed the paper-thin wafer in outstretched hands and spoke the words, 'The body of Christ, broken for you', I felt as if I had been emptied out and as if, in some indefinable way, I was caught up in the midst of that mystical encounter.

The Lord's Table is the place to which we are drawn, the place where we encounter God and are equipped to live life in all its fullness. It's where we participate in the drama of Christ's death, the descent into the darkness of Hades which precedes the return to the light and life. Through the bread and wine, the sacrament of the Eucharist symbolizes the mysterious cycle of death and resurrection. It is the same cycle that is also symbolically enacted in Baptism by our immersion into the watery depths and the rising up into new life.

In my local Anglican church, the sacrament of Baptism is signified by the pouring of water, but in the Baptist church where I grew up the immersion was total. In the church building that I attended as a child, the baptism pool was located beneath the wooden flooring in front of an imposing raised pulpit. During a baptism service, a pool of deep-blue water would be revealed and the candidate would walk down a set of steps into it. Then, standing with their arms crossed before them, they would lie back into the water supported by the minister – an immersion not dissimilar to that carried out by John the Baptist in the waters of the River Jordan.

As a child I was mesmerized by the idea that while we sang and prayed, beneath our feet lay those waters, inviting submersion – an ever-present invitation into the cycle of death and life. And, over the years of cancer, I have often reflected on the truth, embodied in the sacraments of Communion and Baptism, that in one way or another we all have to plumb the shadowy depths – by facing up to our doubts, fears or even our own mortality – before we can be brought back up into the light.

Now the rector brings this mystery into my home and, as he lifts the cup and blesses the bread, we pray together:

Lord, I am not worthy to receive you
But only say the word, and I shall be healed.[2]

As he places the communion wafer in my mouth, I feel once again a profound sense of connection with the drama of Jesus' descent into darkness and his rising up. At the same time, I am acutely conscious of taking into myself the Christ who not only surrounds me but through the indwelling of the Holy

Spirit also somehow mystically exists within me. In the ritual of Communion, I recognize with amazement the pattern of descent into the waters, the encounter with the divine in the depths, followed by a rising back up into the light. I recognize in the sacraments and the spiritual disciplines surrounding them a gateway into a deeper connection with the God whose nature is beyond our imagination; the God who cradled me on the ocean floor.

So, with renewed fervour, I begin each morning in prayer, joining in with the beautiful liturgy of the Daily Office, and reflect on his word, a practice which Benedictines see as a pathway into a deep meditative experience of God. Then, in the silence of the empty house, I fold my broken body and sit cross-legged on my sickbed and focus on my God-given breath, seeking that liminal space of connection. Relentless thoughts continue to intrude but, day by day, I become less attached to them and gradually I find that I'm able to muffle the voice of my internal narrator and sit in alert stillness, waiting on the Lord. I find great peace in the mindfulness of the moment, a sense of liberation at no longer having to wonder about the future.

I realize that I have reached a place of acceptance of the brokenness of my body and am daily filled with gratitude for the simple fact that I am still alive – for the breath in my lungs and my presence in the world – but it still feels as if I'm playing in the shallows. I want to go deeper than this awareness of bodily sensations and the beauty of breath, and yearn to reach beyond the peace of the present to something ancient and eternal that exists in the depths. So, I turn again to the experiences of the early Christians.

The idea of focusing on a single word or collection of words prevails in many Christian contemplative traditions, and is reflected today in some churches in the practice of singing simple worship sings repetitively, reciting words or phrases as a way to focus on God and open ourselves to the presence of the Holy Spirit.

Back in the fifth century, John Cassian, that remarkable recorder of the practices and spirituality of the Desert Fathers, recounted the monks' repetition of a single verse of Scripture or 'formula' which led to the 'renunciation of all riches of thought and imagination'.[3] According to Cassian, the most popular of these prayers was the Jesus Prayer which the Fathers repeated within their minds hundreds of times throughout the day until it became as natural and spontaneous as breathing. This practice was known as 'the prayer of the heart'.

The monastic focus on what might be called a 'mantra', or a one-word prayer, was also developed in *The Cloud of Unknowing* into a programme for would-be fourteenth-century contemplatives. The unknown author advised that, 'We should pray in the height and depth, the length and breadth of our spirit . . . not in many words, but in a little word of one syllable.'[4] He also recommends that the chosen word should be as short as possible, such as GOD or LOVE, as 'short prayers pierce heaven'.[5] Then, when we have chosen our word, he says: 'fasten this word to your heart, so that it never parts from it, whatever happens. This word is to be your shield and your spear, whether you ride in peace or in war. With this word you are to beat on the cloud and darkness above you. With this word you are to hammer down every kind of thought beneath the cloud of forgetting.'[6]

This practice of prayer that goes beyond imagination and words – the prayer that simply seeks to be in the presence of God – was enshrined in the Benedictine rule of life as *oratio pura* or 'pure prayer' – a form of prayer that does not involve thinking about God, imagining ourselves into the holy narrative (as in Ignatian spirituality), or even talking to God; it's about simply *being* in the presence of the one who is beyond thought. This is the approach to prayer which Bede Griffiths and others found their way to via eastern spiritual traditions.

One of those other spiritual masters was the Benedictine monk John Main (1926–82), whom Griffiths regarded as one of the great spiritual guides in the contemporary church. Main, like Griffiths, walked an unconventional path to faith. While serving in the British Colonial Service in Malaysia in the 1950s, Main was introduced to the idea of meditation by a respected Tamil Indian named Swami Satyanda. One afternoon the young officer was drawn into a discussion with him on the subject of prayer. He was so impressed by the spiritual discipline of Satyanda, who meditated twice daily at six o'clock in the morning and evening, that he asked if he, a Christian, could also learn to meditate. Satyanda laughed and replied that, of course, it would only make him a better Christian.[7]

Main took his advice about meditation, which turned out to be disarmingly straightforward; he instructed Main to choose a word or 'mantra' and to just repeat it faithfully throughout two daily periods of meditation. In his meetings with Satyanda Main asked all the usual questions voiced by novice meditators. Am I doing this right? How long will it take for this to work? But each week he was given the same advice: 'Say your mantra.'

The sheer simplicity appealed deeply to Main and after he left Malaysia he continued to meditate for many years. Until, after a university teaching post in Dublin, an unsuccessful marriage proposal and the death of a beloved nephew, he made the decision to join a Benedictine monastery in Ireland. Main was not a conventional candidate and met with a great deal of resistance to his 'eastern' views, and for ten years was forced to give up the practice of meditation. But eventually he went on to teach meditation, first in London and later in Montreal, and to found the World Community for Christian Meditation.

One of the pivotal moments on his journey was the discovery of John Cassian's *Conferences* and his reference to the Desert Fathers' practice of repeating a single verse or formula, which Main related to his own experience of meditation as shaped by his Malaysian teacher. This led to further exploration of the ancient Christian monastic traditions, and Main began to see a profound connection between Cassian's writing, the Benedictine use of the Jesus Prayer, and the writings of the fourteenth-century mystic in *The Cloud of Unknowing*. Drawing on these antecedents, and his own experience, he then formulated his own teaching on contemporary Christian meditation.

Like the early Christian meditators, Main instructed would-be meditators to use a single word or phrase as their 'mantra', or prayer, and recommended the use of the word *Maranatha*, which in Aramaic (the language that Jesus spoke) means 'Come, O Lord'. One of the earliest Christian prayers, the appeal 'Maranatha', appears in Paul's first letter to the Corinthians (16:22) which speaks 'about the indwelling of the human consciousness of Christ in the heart of the believer',[8] and Main describes the mantra as 'like a plough that goes through your mind pushing everything else aside'[9] and a means of entering into the 'resonant harmony of God'.[10] For Main, the purpose of the meditation, and the mantra, is to enable a place of retreat from the distraction of our lives, where we can quieten our thoughts and focus solely on God. By engaging in this form of spiritual discipline, we create the space to simply be in his presence and for the Holy Spirit to work in us. 'The mantra takes up where language fails. It is like God's harmonic.'[11]

Main taught that when meditating one should wear loose comfortable clothing, be seated on a chair or a cushion, and adopt a sitting posture in which you are able to remain completely and utterly still, pointing out that:

> by not moving, by staying still, we will undergo what may perhaps be our first lesson in transcending desires and overcoming that fixation that we so often have with ourselves . . . Then you close your eyes gently and begin to repeat your word – *Maranatha*. The purpose of repeating the word is to gently lead you away from your own thoughts, your own ideas, your own desire, your own sin, and to lead you into the presence of God. Say the word gently, but deliberately, say the word in a relaxed way but articulate it silently in your mind, *Ma – ra – na – tha*. Gradually, as you continue to meditate, the word will sink down into your heart.[12]

His key rule is that, at least at first, one must continue to recite the chosen word throughout the entire period of meditation, and that whenever we are distracted by thoughts or sensations, we must gently bring our mind back to the word, as one does with the breath in mindfulness.

Based on his experience, Main taught that 'the day will come when the mantra ceases to sound and we are lost in the eternal silence of God', but that 'the clear rule is that as soon as we consciously realize that we are in this state of profound silence and begin to reflect about it, we must gently and quietly return to our mantra'.[13] Over time – and for some of us years – the silences become more prolonged, and 'by the stillness in the spirit we move in the ocean of God'.[14] One simply has to persevere in saying the mantra.

As I learn more about John Main's approach to meditation, I am mesmerized by one particular passage of writing in which he likens the reality of God to the sea, and ourselves to figures standing on a far shore:

> Some sit, like King Canute, ordering the tide to turn back. Others gaze romantically at its beauty and vastness from a safe distance. But we are called to be baptized, to be plunged into it, to allow its all-powerful tide to direct our lives . . . The poverty and the joy of our word leads us into the sea and, once there, it keeps us simply in the current of the Spirit that leads us to a place unknown to us, where we know ourselves in him, in his eternal now.
>
> (From: John Main: *Letters from the Heart*.
> The Crossroad Publishing Company)[15]

I take the plunge.

Main stipulates that you should meditate for twenty to thirty minutes early in the morning and in the evening, but I quickly realize that this is not realistic. I'm not a Benedictine monk whose entire life is focused around prayer and, as far as I know, Main didn't have to badger his teenager to get in the shower each morning and check that they are equipped for school before they dash out the door. I also find that as the day progresses my energy levels deplete and the chemotherapy fog rolls in so that, by the time I get to around six o'clock in the evening, I am in danger of dozing off if I sit still for even a few moments. While the state of consciousness that one seeks through meditation is perhaps closer to a dream state than our waking lives (in that you occasionally dip a toe in the water of your unconscious), it does require a state of alertness and 'mindfulness'.

I decide that my initial commitment will be to incorporate twenty minutes of meditation into my existing morning spiritual disciplines. It's quite a commitment as I already spend well over an hour in prayer and reading Scripture, but cancer has ironically granted me the gift of time. *The Cloud of Unknowing* refers to periods of meditation as the 'time of work', so perhaps I've been given this time exactly so that I can engage in this labour.

Once the house empties in the morning, I settle myself cross-legged, a position that is becoming harder to adopt as the treatment goes on but which I still prefer to use for prayer, rather than sitting in a chair (perhaps a residual habit from my time studying in India and Thailand). I first spend time with Scripture, following the Benedictine tradition, in which active engagement with God's word is seen as a stepping stone towards a deeper, wordless encounter with him in the stillness of our souls. I read the sacred words slowly, rolling them over in my mind, allowing them to settle within me, becoming part of a wordless prayer of the heart. Then I close my eyes and silently allow the words of the simple prayer *Maranatha* – 'Come, O Lord' – to rise in my awareness, repeating it gently, faithfully and at times relentlessly.

Ma-ra-na-tha. I sound out the syllables in my mind and soon find that the word seems to synchronize with my breath as in my mindfulness practice. This is to be expected, but I obediently draw my focus away from the sensations of the breath and back to the word. *Ma-ra-na-tha*. The syllables begin to rise and fall like the cresting and falling of waves: *Ma* rising on the wave, *ra* falling, *na* rising and *tha* falling, repeating endlessly, day by day.

As I first start to meditate this way, the word seems to oscillate; sometimes it seems distant, a whisper on the horizon, but at other times it's so close that it occupies the whole of my consciousness but, even then, I'm unable to shut off the flow of images and thoughts. St Theresa of Avila once likened the mind to a ship whose mutinous crew have tied up the captain and are taking turns to steer the boat, first in one direction and then another. And as I seek to once again reach the depths, my own renegade thoughts keep drawing me back to the surface of the water. Just occasionally I am gifted with an insight that seems almost profound, which makes me yearn to record them to share at some later date. Instead, I try to let them go, and return to the word. *Ma-ra-na-tha*.

Frequently, I catch myself chasing after thoughts that are insignificant and trite: remembrance of tasks left undone and random memories that lead me on a merry dance. I become lost in thought, and minutes go by before I realize that I have strayed; frustrated at the wilful chatter of my mind, I then draw my attention back: *Ma-ra-na-tha*. Sometimes I simply feel bored by the incessant repetition and, on occasions, I become distracted by the sensations in my body – an itch in the middle of my back, a nerve twitching in my toes which have gone numb from sitting in one position. At times like these I wonder why on earth I am even doing this, but remind myself of the advice within *The Cloud of Unknowing* that:

Anyone who habitually practises this work will unquestionably find it laborious, yes, very laborious indeed . . . the labour is all in treading down the thoughts of all beings that God ever created, and in keeping them beneath the cloud of forgetting . . . Then perhaps he will at times send out a beam of spiritual light, piercing this cloud of unknowing that is between you and him, and show you some of his mysteries, of which human beings are not permitted or able to speak. Then you will sense your feelings aflame with the fire of his love.[16]

The reason I am doing this is to seek that intuitive connection with God; to feel once again his profound presence – and if I can recreate something of the experience I had with him on the ocean floor it will be worth it. So, I return to the task and repeat the word – *Ma-ra-na-tha* – until gradually, almost imperceptibly, something changes and, between the rising and the falling of the prayer, I detect not the sound of my own thoughts but that blessed silence, and that profound stillness. It's as if, by keeping my rational mind occupied on the surface, the repetition has allowed me access to a different, deeper level of intuitive consciousness, the place of meeting with the one whose nature is beyond language or imagination.

There I wait, in anticipation,

in the belief that something hidden will manifest.

Until once again in deep waters

I find myself standing on the crest of a great ocean shelf.

Gazing out into a blue abyss

to that eternal mystery that lies beyond.

And in the stillness, I feel him

around me, within me,

closer than my own breath.
In union with every being,
pervading the universe.

The experience is only transitory, and in the moment of recognition the connection slips away and my mind is once again
in motion – *Ma-ra-na-tha* – but just for a moment the cloud
is pierced and, in that place of wonder, I'm no longer conscious of my thoughts, but of a vast unending ocean of love.
In going deeper into my own consciousness, I seem to have
found the God that exists both beyond but also within.

Part Three

Arrival

24

Black Dog

For the first time in months, I feel as if I've reached that spacious place spoken of in the Psalms and, from this vantage point, I dare to look into the future – to a time beyond cancer. This journey has been so unpredictable, with so many unexpected twists and turns, that I've tried not to think more than a few days or weeks ahead in order to avoid disappointment and disillusionment. Now, for the first time, I'm emboldened to imagine a future in which I am actually included – trusting in God's plans to give me hope and a future. But just as I begin to dare to look down the path ahead, I am once again knocked off course.

I'm woken in the middle of the night by crippling pains in my abdomen. It feels as if I am being stabbed repeatedly in the belly with a carving knife until I want to vomit. I try to get out of bed but find I am unable to stand, so crawl over the carpet towards the bathroom door. As I kneel by the toilet basin, my whole body repeatedly goes into spasm, hour after hour, until all I can do is lie on the cold stone floor, drained, exhausted and scared.

At five o'clock in the morning, I stop being ill long enough to call the oncology nurse, who once again tells me to go straight to A&E. I wake John, who has decamped to the spare room during my treatment in an effort to insulate me from the bugs that circulate in school. He helps me stagger to the car and, as the sun creeps over the horizon, we drive the familiar route to the hospital. As the hedgerows roll by, I realize I am crying – not howling sobs, but a gentle rain of tears.

Once we arrive, John goes off in search of a wheelchair and eventually we get into reception. I'm seen immediately by the triage nurse, who takes me straight round to a side ward. Given that Covid is still circulating, John is sent away and a nurse is dispatched to try to get some fluids into my severely dehydrated body. After ten minutes of stabbing away at my arm, she informs me once again that the veins in my arm and hand are wrecked, but eventually she manages to insert a cannula into the inside of my wrist, tearing the vein in the process.

By this point I have stopped being sick, and the stabbing pain in my stomach is now more bearable, so I convince myself that I've just had an unfortunate reaction to the latest round of chemo and bio-targeted treatments. I'm therefore taken by surprise when a surgeon arrives, examines my X-rays, probes my abdomen – sending me into paroxysms of pain – and tells me: 'We think you may have a bowel obstruction which is now perforated and we need to prep you for emergency surgery.'

Blind panic ensues: 'Emergency surgery! Wait, I can't have surgery – I have to have the next chemo. I can't stop the chemo; I've got an aggressive cancer! We can't do this.'

The surgeon is not moved and bluntly points out, 'If it's bowel perforation we can't leave you like this as you'll be dead within a week.'

I am stunned into silence. I thought things were looking up; I seemed to be tolerating the chemotherapy better and had dared to look ahead. The surgeon disappears and I'm left to contemplate the implications of a delay in the cancer treatment. For the next hour and a half, I lie in my cubicle praying; the stillness and the calm of the previous weeks now seem like a distant memory as fear breaks through and overwhelms me.

I realize with startling clarity that I *really* don't want to die, and certainly not like this. Surely, I can't end up dying simply because I couldn't go to the loo! It would be a ludicrous and ignoble way to shuffle off this mortal coil. Unfortunate images of Elvis dying on the toilet flash through my mind and I lie there wallowing in self-pity, quietly snivelling like a child, and wondering how on earth this latest crisis squares with God's plans to prosper me and to give me hope and a future. My reading of this scriptural gift has been that God was reassuring me that I will once again survive cancer, but I realize now that the future he speaks of could refer to the afterlife. Perhaps I have misinterpreted his intentions. *Could it actually be God's will to let me die?*

An hour into the wait, a nurse puts her head around the curtain to check on me. Spotting the cross in my hand she asks if I am a Christian. I nod mutely and she tells me that she's a Catholic, and that one of her dearest wishes is to go on retreat in Bethlehem. In the chaos of A&E we talk about the Holy Land and I show her my clutch cross made from olive wood from the birthplace of Christ. As she turns to go, she smiles broadly and encourages me: 'You keep on holding on to that – he will bring you through.' It feels as if God has sent her to restore my equilibrium and, by the time she leaves, the storm within me has begun to subside and I fall into a restless sleep.

It's almost midday when I feel a gentle hand on my arm. It's the surgeon again, who tells me that he's discussed my case with a senior surgeon, and they are now confident that I don't require emergency surgery and I can go home. I can hardly believe it. Over the past few hours, I have been to hell and back imagining how such surgery would impact my cancer treatment and now I'm being sent home. I am both delighted and bewildered.

Back at home, I find I am unsettled. Something about the experience has shaken my foundations, so much so that I'm hardly surprised when my oncologist contacts me to say that he is concerned that this might be a sign that the cancer has spread. He goes on to say that it may be necessary to halt the chemotherapy and move quickly on with the mastectomy, in order to clear the way for dealing with this new problem. As a first step, he says he will arrange further investigations, including a CT scan to see if there is any sign of cancer in the colon and to assess how effectively the chemotherapy has attacked the original cancer.

As the call comes to an end, the seriousness of my situation comes back to me with full force. Over the past couple of months, I've been so absorbed and even excited by what God seems to be teaching me on this journey that I have almost forgotten why I was forced to set out in the first place. Despite the ongoing impact of the treatment, I'd been so focused on where God seemed to be leading me that the cancer itself had been relegated to the back of my mind. Taking to heart Jesus' admonition against 'babbling like pagans [who] think they will be heard because of their many words' (Matthew 6:7), I had stopped coming to him with prayers about specific steps on my journey or detailed requests for healing. Rather, I had trusted in Christ's assurance that our Father knows what we need before we ask him. As I had gone deeper into contemplation, I had been trying to keep my sights firmly fixed on the Healer rather than his healing, surrendering to him and praying 'Thy Will Be Done'. Now the seriousness of my situation has come to the fore again – *I have recurrent aggressive cancer! How could I have been so distracted from this reality?*

I continue to try to meditate, but my thoughts are now much more intrusive. I try to force them down with the mantra, but two mental states seem to be battling against each other – one of peace, the other of fear. As I sit in meditation, I am conscious only of my body throbbing with pain and my veins burning within me. It's as if the chemotherapy is gnawing away whatever health and vitality is left within me. I try to view my broken body without judgment, with acceptance, but now my soul feels leaden, weighed down with all the worry that I thought I had handed over to God. No matter how much I try, I can no longer find the stillness, and I am plagued by the suspicion that I may be slipping into depression.

As a young woman, one of my main fears was that I had inherited my father's mental health issues. My childhood was a wonderful one but a roller-coaster experience, as my father swung between periods of euphoric creativity and severe depression. When at the height of good mood, my father was a brilliant and witty raconteur, loved by all, but as he descended into depression he became like a black vortex which threatened to pull us all into the darkness of his inner world. Early on, my mother and sister seemed to find a way to insulate themselves against this gravitational pull, but I was more susceptible, and as my father went down I would also be dragged into the depths of despair and grief for him. I found it heartbreaking to see him suffer so much.

He always used to say that he could see too much of himself in me, which is perhaps why we were so close and he chose to share his despair with me. It was a terrible burden that he put on such young shoulders and, when I left home, I hoped that it might become lighter. Perhaps subconsciously that's why I moved to Wales to study – I needed to put the mountains between us. However, my adoration of my father, and the dread, followed me first to Aberystwyth and then to London, where one Monday morning at work I received a telephone call from him telling me that he was going to kill himself.

Mercifully, he didn't actually follow through on the threat, but that day something inside me broke. I felt so helpless; I was 60 miles away and could do nothing to stop my father from taking his own life, or to lift the despair that drove him to contemplate such a dreadful act. I don't remember a great deal about the subsequent events (there's a week of my life that is erased from my memory) but my housemates later told me I'd informed them – ironically in hindsight – that I had cancer, before barricading myself in the house, leaving them standing in the street in Muswell Hill. What I do remember is being told by a psychiatrist that I had suffered a mental breakdown. Her theory was that the breakdown had been a long time coming and was born out of the overwhelming sense of responsibility I had felt for my father from a very young age – a reversal of the natural pattern of parent–child relations. I was not bipolar and didn't even have clinical depression; I had just broken under the weight of love for my father.

I rejected the proffered antidepressants but spent some valuable months in therapy and eventually normal service resumed. However, the incident seemed to leave a crack in my psyche which the darkness would occasionally creep through.

My father used to call his inner shadow the 'black dog' and, in the years following, I would sometimes find that my own dark canine would appear out of nowhere, like a storm cloud that blocks out the sun. Sometimes there was an incident that triggered the melancholy, but on other occasions the 'black dog' seemed to come of its own volition, triggering emotions that were out of step with my circumstances. At times like these I tended to try to count my blessings but, as most people with depression will tell you, this doesn't always help (in fact it's about as helpful as being told to 'buck up'). The reality is that it's perfectly possible to be profoundly grateful for all the things that God has blessed you with – love, family, security, health – but still feel overwhelmed by this sense of ennui.

As Christians, we can sometimes labour under the impression that if we are not continually joyful then we have failed to have sufficient faith. But while the Bible doesn't include the word 'depression', there are various key players in God's narrative who are variously described as 'downcast', 'broken-hearted', 'troubled', 'despairing' and 'miserable'. Jonah, for example, once cried out that he was 'angry enough to die' (Jonah 4:9); Elijah wailed, 'I have had enough, Lord', and pleaded, 'Take my life' (1 Kings 19:4); and Jeremiah lamented, 'Cursed be the day I was born! . . . Why did I ever come out of the womb to see trouble and sorrow and to end my days in shame?' (Jeremiah 20:14,18). Even Jesus, when facing the hour of his crucifixion, admitted to his disciples, 'My soul is overwhelmed with sorrow to the point of death' (Mark 14:34). Now, like so many others down the centuries, I too cry out the words of the psalmist: 'Why are you downcast, O my soul?' (Psalm 42:5).

It isn't only the ever-present threat of death that has brought me low; that has hung over my head for nearly eight years now and I have faced up to the lurking fear, wrestled with it and to some extent subdued it. The reality is that I'm not afraid of death itself as I'm utterly convinced to the depths of my being that death is not the end. The rational journalist within me is convinced of this by two key pieces of evidence. First, the prevalence of belief in some form of afterlife in nearly every single culture since the dawn of humankind (it's as if the knowledge that this life is not the end is hardwired into every soul on earth), and second, the fact of the resurrection.

The claim that Jesus was raised from the dead is of course the most outrageous claim of all, but the one on which my hope, and that of 2.7 billion people, is based. Greater minds than mine have spent centuries dissecting the historical accounts of the resurrection in the gospels of Matthew, Mark, Luke and John, as well as the non-canonical *Gospel of Peter*, all of which include eyewitness accounts of sightings of the risen Christ. But there are a number of factors that have led to my firm personal belief in the authenticity of these accounts. For example, if the gospels were a well-constructed piece of false propaganda, why would disciples have recorded that the first people to see the risen figure of Jesus were women, when their gender rendered their testimony invalid in the first century? And, perhaps most convincingly of all, why on earth would the disciples have been willing to put themselves in such danger to promote this claim if they knew it was a lie – a path that for many ended in the most appalling deaths? It just doesn't make any sense. So, rationally, I concluded that the only explanation could be that Jesus really did rise from the dead, no matter how fantastical that might seem.

My conviction, however, isn't one only of the head but also of the heart. Having heard my mother's testimony of her experiences at the point of her passing – and having been with her at the moment of her death – I am utterly convinced that, in some intangible way, she lives on. As her body failed, it was as if her spirit burned more brightly and, as she took her last breath, I had the distinct impression that her spirit had left her body and moved on. Since then, no rational argument or fearmongering can take away her deathbed legacy. It was as if the veil between heaven and earth was lifted for a short while, and that moment has transformed my belief about our reality for ever.

This doesn't mean, however, that my cancer hasn't caused great sadness. At times I have been overwhelmed with grief at the thought of having to leave my darling husband and beloved children. They are my world and I would gladly lay down my life for each and every one of them if I thought it would save them. But I cannot see any sense in my death from cancer – no saving grace. It would only break their hearts and leave their lives fractured and incomplete. I cannot bear the idea of my husband facing the rest of his life alone. He has always been a bit of a loner (I sometimes have to remind my-self that before he met me, John had happily spent a year and a half cycling round Australia on his own – a clear indication of his self-sufficiency), but we have found great joy living our lives together while respecting each other's independence. Our family means everything to my darling John, and I can see the toll that the uncertainty of cancer has taken on him.

It's also too painful to even contemplate how my death would impact my children; my eldest is just finding her feet in the world and my youngest is in that critical transition period from adolescence to early independence. I'm sure the security and stability of their family, knowing that there is a home they can always retreat to, and a mother and father who are always there with open arms, has helped them find their way. I can't bear to think what it would do to them if that stability were to be shaken. It breaks my heart to think of the scars carried throughout life by children who are robbed of a parent too early.

On my better days I'm able to keep such sad thoughts at bay, but the relentlessness of the treatments is slowly taking its toll, wearing me down. With each treatment I become physically weaker, and with each onslaught my robustness of spirit and God-given mental resilience seems to be eroded. As my natural optimism begins to fade, I enter a state of melancholy which saps my strength.

I also begin to feel lonely for the first time. I know that there are so many people out there who have to face the challenge of cancer alone and I feel ashamed at giving way to the emotion. I also know that I am so blessed by my beloved family, who are doing all they can to support me, encourage me and comfort me. But it is, of course, possible to feel alone even when in the midst of a crowd. Our pain, internal struggles, fears and suffering are ours alone – hermetically sealed within our biology. No matter how close we may feel to our nearest and dearest, they can never see the world through our eyes – nor can we through theirs. We come into, and leave, the world alone, and the harsh reality is that, on our journey between life and death, there's no one on earth that can truly share in our experiences, good or bad – except for the God who dwells within us, and knows the deepest unspoken yearnings of our heart – but this doesn't stop our yearning for connection.

Until now, I have been almost savouring my seclusion as the rest of the world get on with their lives, and have recognized the value of my enforced 'retreat', but I now realize how truly isolated I am. Covid is still with us but, as the vaccination programme rolls out, life for the vast majority of people has begun to return to some kind of normality. While I cower behind closed doors avoiding a virus which, given my lack of immunity, could prove deadly, others are out in the world, doing those things that we formerly took for granted: going shopping, meeting up with friends and taking beach holidays. I have no resentment – I do not begrudge them these simple joys of life – but the reality is that the loosening of restrictions for the majority has simply tightened the bonds for that group now known as the 'clinically extremely vulnerable'.

Zoom and FaceTime have helped me to retain some connection to the world and I have been very blessed by the willingness of my sister and other close friends to take the necessary tests and sit in the garden with me, rain or shine. However, I still feel separated from the community at large, in particular my church family, and now, in my melancholy, I seem to retreat even further away from the world. I stop messaging or phoning friends, avoid Zoom calls and sink further into myself. Since the onset of treatment, I've written a blog called *Faith, Life and Cancer* and posted on social media about all that God is teaching me on this cancer journey, but now I struggle to find the words: I am ashamed of my emotional state which feels like a failure of faith, even though I know that this is a misnomer.

Then a tiny miracle occurs, another one of those little synchronicities or God-incidences in life that leave you wondering. In this case it's a small thing, a simple direct message on Facebook from a friend who used to be on my team at World Vision UK. We'd only had very limited contact since she'd left to take up a new job in another part of the country, but then one Sunday morning, when I am lost in my own darkness, I receive a message from her:

> Kate. You've been on my mind the past couple of days and I've been praying for you. I felt to pray against 'the dark night of the soul'. The 'dark nights' are the moments/days when even though we have huge faith and confidence in God's power, the things of this world just get very overwhelming. So I was praying that however you're feeling, you'd be very, very aware of God's presence. That's the thing that carries us through the worst that life throws our way.

It's only a very small miracle but I know that, through my friend, God is telling me to hold on and to have faith that he *is* the God of miracles, Jehovah Rapha; that he has plans to give me hope and a future and, if I hold on to this, he will draw me out of this darkness and back into the light.

I reflect back on the last few months and begin to see a pattern. The scriptures that seemed to reach me just at the point when I needed them most; from God's promise in Jeremiah 29 which found its way to me at the outset of this journey, to the psalms that articulated the deepest cries of my soul when I could find no words. The encounters with others as I have traversed this harsh terrain; from the extraordinary Christ-like compassion of the caregivers of the NHS, to fellow patients whom God seemed to bring me into contact with so that I could encourage them; from the prayerful nurse who appeared at my side like a ministering angel, to the friends who have helped me in my time of need. There's the tangible presence that I experienced in the depths of my illness – my ocean floor experience – and the books and other writings recommended to me by friends and my spiritual director that have helped me to find meaning in the depths and opened me up to a new intuitive relationship with God.

The theologian and cancer patient Ken Curtis once said: 'Being weak and wounded in spirit does not have to mean that we are finished. It could mean that we are on the verge of a new beginning. A place where our heart can open to that which far exceeds anything we have seen or known before.'[1] Didn't Jesus tell us, 'Blessed are the poor in spirit' (Matthew 5:3)? Perhaps it's only when our spirit is broken that we can truly comprehend the miraculous, so I continue to pray and to meditate.

Every day, I force myself out of my despondency to lift up my incoherent and confused prayers, seeking solace in God's word; and seeking him in the silence of my heart, I try to pierce the cloud of my own melancholy and find the miracle of his presence. I use the mantra like a great rock, forcing down the self-pity and fear that threatens to engulf me. *Ma-ra-na-th-a, Ma-ra-na-tha-a.* I wield the word like a battering ram against the door that seems to separate me from God, knocking with all my might, trusting in Jesus' promise that if we knock, the door will be opened (Matthew 7:7), and that if I continue seeking, I will find him, the Alpha and the Omega, Elohim, Adonai, the source of all being, Jehovah Rapha, the God who heals the world and all humankind.

Stubbornly, doggedly, I persist, conscious of the need to somehow get beyond my conscious self and my meandering thoughts, emotions and mental images. I try not to be disheartened by my apparent inability to meditate, and hold on to John Main's advice not to judge one's facility as either good or bad but to always, simply, return to the mantra.

Ma-ra-na-tha, Ma-ra-na-tha. It almost becomes part of me; a rhythm as steady as my heart, beating in the depth of my being.

Gradually I find it easier to part my thoughts in order to detect that majestic stillness beyond and, in doing so, it's as if I am piercing the clouds of my own melancholy, finding a type of peace. Perhaps it's because I am no longer focusing my attention on myself and my insignificant fears but on the something infinitely greater than I can even imagine and, in doing so, my perspective has altered. When we praise, it opens a door in our heart to the awesome and mysterious nature of God, and our own troubles pale into insignificance.

Until one day, once again, I catch a glimpse. It's only a momentary glance but, for a short while, the waters of my mind are becalmed. In the stillness I become conscious of something indefinable, indescribable, and eternal, that lies beyond but also within, and I am lost in wonder and praise.

25

Trust Fall

So, I go to the hospital for yet another CT scan. As I disappear into the doughnut-like scanning machine, I close my eyes, clutch my cross and begin to say a silent prayer, and, as I do so, a memory rises up of a game that I used to play at school called the Trust Fall. It's one of the traditional playground amusements that predates the technology that now so occupies kids, in which a child stands within a ring of their fellow pupils, allowing themselves to fall backwards, testing their belief in whether or not they will be caught by their peers.

This game, which is now sometimes used as part of corporate team building, was really popular when I was in middle school and I remember, on more than one occasion, finding my trust was misplaced as I toppled backwards unsupported onto the concrete playground floor. But more often, I felt the arms of friendship catch me and guide me gently to the ground. I think the main lesson I learned from the whole exercise was: be careful who you trust! As I pray, I am reminded of this game.

The reality is that my medical situation has become so complex that I don't actually know what to pray for any more. So, as my certainty gives way beneath me, I lie in the scanner and pray. *Lord, I just don't know, but I also know that I don't need to know. I am just going to hand all this over to you. You know what is best in a way that I never can, so I place my whole life in your hands. 'Thy kingdom come, Thy will be done in earth, as it is in heaven'* (Matthew 6:10 KJV).

Many of us will find times in our lives when our challenges seem so complex that we struggle to know what supplications to make to God on our own behalf, or on behalf of others – and this is particularly true when it comes to healing. Certainly, my own situation has become far too complicated to fully comprehend. I'm not a doctor but, as I lie in wait, I realize that I don't need to be. I don't need to understand every medical nuance or to be able to pray for specific outcomes or procedures. I just need to trust.

It's not that I am renouncing responsibility; I will certainly make sure that I know enough to ask all the right questions when I go to meet the medics, but I realize that I don't need to have all the answers. Because when we pray, we are reaching out to one who created every particle, atom, cell and organ in our bodies:

> For you created my inmost being;
>> you knit me together in my mother's womb.
> I praise you because I am fearfully and wonderfully made;
>> your works are wonderful,
>> I know that full well.
> My frame was not hidden from you
>> when I was made in the secret place.
> When I was woven together in the depths of the earth,
>> your eyes saw my unformed body.
> All the days ordained for me
>> were written in your book
>> before one of them came to be.

Psalm 139:13–16

It was God's extraordinary imagination that created the spark that brought matter into being and enabled the development of life in all its complexity. He knows the answers – and this is something I can surrender control to. I also reflect on Larry Dossey's point that non-directive 'Thy Will Be Done' prayers seem to be just as effective – or even more effective – than the kind of directive prayers for specific outcomes that we are more familiar with. Trust, it seems, lies at the core of healing. So, faced with the complexity of my own body and the multiplicity of medical diagnoses, I once again let go, trusting in God to catch me and to do what is best for me.

A week later I meet my oncologist who tells me that the investigations show that the cancer hasn't spread. He goes on to say, 'In fact, the chemotherapy has worked so well that two of the tumours have halved in size and the third has completely melted away. You have a performance level of zero.'

'Is that good?'

'It is the best possible result!'

I grin at him like a small child and want to hug him. But the person I really want to hug is God. *Thy will be done.*

The next step is to meet the surgeon to discuss options. There are still two more cycles of chemotherapy to go but it's time to begin planning the next phase of my treatment. Earlier on in the process, I had undertaken the recommended BRCA test to check if I had the 'breast cancer gene'. The decision to take the test was not an easy one; it's a little like opening Pandora's box as once you have taken this step there is no going back. Once you have the knowledge, it can't be put back in the box, and you and your loved ones have to learn how to live with it. I've never had a desire to know what the future may hold, eschewing horoscopes and other kinds of fortune-telling, working on the basis that knowing what lies ahead would take the adventure out of living.

If you have children, the decision is even more difficult, because that knowledge affects not only your own future but that of the next generation, leaving them to struggle with the implications, and often the need to make seemingly impossible decisions of their own. The test, however, also opens up the potential to control that future to some extent. If you are found to carry the gene, then you, and your offspring, can access monitoring at a much earlier age, allowing for the early detection that saves lives. As such, the decision in the end was easy. Given that my grandmother died of breast cancer in her fifties and I've now had cancer twice in three different varieties, taking the test seemed the only responsible thing to do.

Getting the test itself was simple; what was more difficult was the wait for the phone call to receive the results – which is why the hospital provided a counsellor to talk me through the procedure and its implications for me and my family. When the call finally came, the counsellor asked me if I still wanted to hear the results, before, thankfully, delivering the news that the tests were negative. The relief was enormous.

At around the same time, I had also been to see a plastic surgeon to discuss possible reconstruction. He had laid me out on a gurney, gathered rolls of fat, poked my thighs and then, beaming, informed me that it would be possible to do a single, and at a push, double reconstruction based upon my own tissue. The reconstructed breasts would be smaller than my own, which was a plus as far as I was concerned, and I would get a free tummy tuck thrown in. I could even have it done without temporary implants, although the result would not be as aesthetically pleasing.

He had gone on to explain the procedure, which involved taking 'tissue flaps' from either your tummy, thighs, back or buttocks and using these to create a breast-like shape. It is a complicated procedure that requires the reconnection of blood vessels to create a living replacement, and the surgery takes between eight and eleven hours depending on whether you have a single or double reconstruction. I was also shown photographs of his handiwork which I thought impressive, but when he asked the million-dollar question, 'Why do you want a reconstruction?', I realized that I actually didn't know.

As there were still some months to go before possible surgery, he told me that I could take my time making the decision and sent me away clutching various leaflets. However, a seed of doubt had been planted in my mind and, when I hit the first set of chemotherapy complications, I decided that I didn't want to put my body through any procedure that was not strictly a medical necessity. I fully respect the fact that for others the psychological benefits of retaining your body shape can make this a necessary procedure – particularly if you are younger. But at the age of 58, I had reconciled myself to the idea of having a double mastectomy and then 'living flat' (that is, without any form of reconstruction and even potentially prosthetics). Then, having reached a decision, I had pushed the prospect of surgery to the back of my mind.

The last time I'd seen the surgeon who would carry out my mastectomy was at the very beginning of my cancer journey and, as I enter her office, I cut a rather different and diminished figure. It's painfully evident that the treatments and complications have taken a significant toll on my well-being and, despite my desire to get the whole business over and done with, my surgeon advises me that, given how ill I have been during chemotherapy, she is concerned about putting me through a double mastectomy at this point. My heart sinks.

I explain that I've come to terms with the prospect and believe that I would benefit both psychologically and physically. 'I know that I can't get rid of the risk completely, but I've had three kinds of breast cancer now, and I want to do all I can to reduce the risk of this coming back.'

She listens to me patiently, so I plough on.

'Plus I'm well endowed, you know. If I only have one breast, I'm going to be lopsided and it's going to make my back pain even worse.' *I can't believe that I am trying to persuade a surgeon to cut away extra flesh.*

Having heard me out, she offers reluctantly, 'If you really want me to, I am willing to do it, but there are risks, and these are greater with a double mastectomy – it will be only four weeks after chemo.'

'What kind of risks?'

'The wound not healing, infections, DVTs.' She ticks off the horrors on the fingers of her right hand. 'And there's the risk of your body being cooler for longer – a double takes three to four hours, whereas a single only takes ninety minutes.'

She goes on to explain that, due to the risk created by the pandemic, the hospital is currently managing single mastectomies off site at a private clinic with no overnight facilities and, if I had a double mastectomy, I would need to be taken by ambulance back to the main hospital and admitted to a ward for an overnight stay with potential exposure to Covid. Finally, she points out that they will need to put a wound drain into both sides and as a result I will be fairly incapacitated.

Looking directly at my husband she adds, 'She may even need to be taken to the loo!'

My heart sinks once again. I know that the risk of recurrence can't be eradicated but, in my mind, cutting away the potential had become an imperative. I don't know how to move forward, but then she offers a lifeline when she says, 'You don't carry the BRAC gene but the breast tissue is obviously unstable and a double mastectomy will definitely be in your best interests, so I can do a second surgery six months after radiotherapy.'

The thought of going through two surgeries is daunting and I look hesitant.

'You don't have to make a decision now; go away and think about it.'

As we get up to leave, she adds: 'I promise, from my point of view, I want to give you your life back and not leave you where you are now.'

Before we leave the unit, a care nurse brings out a couple of prosthetics which I weigh in my hands like incongruous silicone blancmanges. They are heavier than I expected and I can see that they would be very convincing. There are certainly members of our church and the local breast cancer group who wear them and, if they hadn't confided in me, I would never have known.

I go away to mull and pray over the decision. Typically, part of me is very keen to get this whole surgery done and dusted, over and done with; I want to draw a line in the sand and to get on with whatever life I have left to live. But an inner voice of wisdom tells me that it would be patently foolhardy to insist on having a double mastectomy in defiance of the

wisdom of the surgeon. Reluctantly I reach a decision. I will
have a single mastectomy to remove the active cancer and a
second mastectomy several months later to reduce the risk of
another recurrence. Once again, I'm having to readjust my
expectations.

I had already reconciled myself to the idea of living flat
without both breasts or any kind of reconstruction, but now,
as I contemplate the journey ahead, I am hit by a sense of
loss; a mastectomy, whether single or double, cuts into the
very sense of a woman's identity. I've never regarded myself
as overtly feminine and my darling husband has repeatedly
reassured me that he really doesn't care what they cut off me
as he simply wants me to keep living.

I tell myself that it isn't as if I am losing an arm or a leg;
the loss of one or both breasts isn't going to disable me – but I
have the nasty feeling I am being pruned. I recall my mother
pruning the rose bushes in our garden at Larkland to the point
where they looked stunted, decapitated and mutilated. In the
winter, the mangled limbs appeared dead and it was hard to
imagine that one day they would burst again into glorious
bloom, petal upon petal, their fragrance filling the air. I know
that many women have faced this reality as part of their cancer
journey, but I still feel daunted by what lies ahead; this process
of pruning the body, the cutting away of cancerous flesh in order to ensure the continuation of life, seems overwhelming –
and, like all serious pruning, I know it's going to hurt.

I also feel as if I am being pruned on a deeper, spiritual
level. The Gospel of John records Jesus telling the disciples
that God 'cuts off every branch in me that bears no fruit, while
every branch that does bear fruit he prunes so that it will be

even more fruitful' (15:2), so perhaps I am being pruned by God. Nevertheless, even if it's the Almighty wielding divine secateurs, pruning is a fairly brutal business. But I tell myself that God doesn't bother pruning branches that don't bear fruit, or are no longer part of the vine.

Jesus himself said: 'I am the vine; you are the branches. If you remain in me and I in you, you will bear much fruit; apart from me you can do nothing. If you do not remain in me, you are like a branch that is thrown away and withers; such branches are picked up, thrown into the fire and burned' (John 15:5–6 NIV 2011). Perhaps it is only those branches that have the potential to bear fruit that he takes the trouble to prune. Pruning may hurt like hell but it isn't a punishment; it's a sign of God's love for us. In order for us to flourish, God has to cut away those parts of our lives that are spiritually dead – the dead flesh; otherwise, rot will set in and spread to other parts of our lives.

I am not yet sure what the result of this pruning – both physical and spiritual – will be, but I'm hopeful that the meaning will emerge. What I do know, however, is that God will use this time in some profound way to his purpose.

26

Anticipation

I head back to the cancer centre for my last chemotherapy treatment. It feels like a very significant moment, although I won't be ringing the bell to signal the end of my treatment quite yet, as I still have twelve months of monoclonal antibody treatments to go. Still, it feels like the beginning of a new chapter.

Ironically, just as I've reached the end of the chemotherapy cycles, I seem to have finally learned how to live with the effects – to be able to accept the roller-coaster ride for what it is. I've grown used to the initial hiatus after each treatment, when it feels as if I'm standing on the top of a vertiginous cliff preparing to leap over the edge into the depths below, anticipating the cool rush of water that will soothe my burning body and ragged mind – followed by descent down through the waters.

While the physical side effects of chemotherapy are still tough, I have over time come to appreciate the space the recovery process creates to simply *be* with God, the disabling effects of chemotherapy keeping me from the relentless round of activity which separates me from the experience of God's presence. Now, as I stand on the cliff's edge for hopefully the last time, I have a sense of anticipation for what God will teach me on this next leg of the journey and a hope that he is preparing me to once again 'declare the works of the LORD' (Psalm 118:17 KJV).

One of the most misunderstood passages in the Bible is Romans 8:28 in which Paul writes: 'in all things God works for the good of those who love him, who have been called according to his purpose.' All too often, this passage is interpreted as a promise that Christians will be somehow spared from suffering; that once you come to Christ, your life will be a bed of roses. In fact, what it means is that God can draw good from even the most challenging experiences of our lives and use them to his purpose. I begin to wonder how God will use this cancer experience for his purpose; whether he will once again take the lemons of my life and make lemonade.

On the morning of my last chemotherapy treatment, *The Bible in One Year* talks about our role as 'Christ's ambassadors' (2 Corinthians 5:20) and the privilege and responsibility of representing Jesus in this world – being God's representatives on earth. The same day, TBN starts to rerun the latest series of my TV show *Living a Transformed Life* and, from the chemo suite, I'm able to post on my blog and social media that, through the wonders of technology, I'll be in two different places that day. That as I sit hooked up to the apparatus of healing in the chemotherapy suite, I'll also be appearing on TV screens, talking about what it means to live a transformed life (albeit with rather more hair, given that the series was filmed prior to my treatment).

When I arrive the chemo suite is very full, buzzing with life, and at first there are no spaces available for me in the medical bays. I wander down through the ward and spot my friend from World Vision who's reading a copy of my latest book *Soul's Scribe*. We sit together and she tells me that my book has helped her to understand how God has worked in her life. When I am summoned and make my way to my allotted treatment chair, I also see someone reading a copy of my memoir *Sea Changed*. I am flabbergasted. Even if my first book was technically a bestselling biography for a while, most books by Christian authors don't exactly flood the market. It feels as if this is one of those meaningful coincidences, a convergence of ideas and encounters that seems to be reinforcing my mission to 'declare the works of the Lord'.

I sit down in a vacant chair by the window and greet my fellow travellers. In one corner sits a neatly dressed elderly lady whose table is laid out with a tray of watercolour blocks and an assortment of brushes. She is utterly absorbed as she paints a study of a flower from a photograph. I ask to see what she is doing and she shows me her work with touching pride. She's obviously enjoying the process enormously and her enjoyment sets the tone for the room. Opposite her sits a middle-aged gentleman who tells me with disarming cheerfulness that he has liver cancer and, in the other corner directly opposite me, a young woman lies on one of the few hospital beds in the suite.

As a nurse connects me to the IV, the patient on the bed props herself up on her elbows, smiles broadly and says, 'I love your turban – where did you find it?' She is much younger than most of the other patients and is so buoyant and animated that it almost feels as if she doesn't belong here. I'm immediately drawn to her like a moth to a flickering flame. We slip into the usual chemo suite patter and she tells me that she has just finished radiotherapy and is on her second weekly chemotherapy cycle. It strikes me as odd that she is being treated in a hospital bed rather than a chair but perhaps it's because the ward is simply so full. She asks me how often I come to the suite and I explain that this is my last actual chemo cycle but that I will continue to come on a three-weekly basis for my monoclonal antibody treatments for another year, adding that I hope to ring the bell next September. She laughs and says, 'I'll take that any day.'

It's the kind of good-natured conversation that I've engaged in so many times before over the past few months of treatment. I ask the usual question: 'What kind of cancer?'

With a smile on her face, she replies, 'Cervical. Terminal. I've got four months.'

I am immediately hit by a surreal sense of dissonance and, speechless, I gaze at this bright, vivacious young woman; the smile is still plastered on her face, but tears now slowly course down her cheek. All I can say is, 'Bless you, bless you, bless you.' I just want to go over and pray for her, but a second sense tells me that this would not be appropriate, so instead I just tell her that I wish I could come over and hug her.

At this point, her young husband arrives at her bedside, takes her hand and sits with her – their love is palpable. I avert my gaze to give them some privacy but am horrified at the thought of them being so cruelly ripped apart before they have really had time to live and learn about each other; to make mistakes and to forgive each other; to face the challenges and joys of sharing their one and only existence with each other; to grow old together. Instead, this young man is going to have to sit beside a hospital bed watching his wife gradually fade away, until this vibrant woman who is so full of life is no more. All that will be left is memories. It seems so

unjust. I close my eyes and pray, *Why, Lord? I don't understand.*
But as I watch them out of the corner of my eye, I'm struck
by how peaceful they both seem. There is something radiant
about them both and I believe that, while it may defy understanding, God is somehow there with them in the midst of
this awful situation.

When I get back home after the last treatment, I begin to
write. The words just pour out of me as if I'm being driven to
record all that God has been showing me. I still have no idea
how the story will end, but I realize that there's a tale I need to
tell; I need to capture the ideas, images and experiences that I
have been granted on this journey, no matter how hard it is to
put some of them into words. And when I don't write, I paint.

It's many years now since I've picked up a paintbrush,
despite spending five years at art school. As a student my
work was largely abstract, but this style was replaced by a
semi-superrealism when I realized that I needed to make some
money and that people would buy paintings of their houses,
children and dogs. But the reality is that while my technical
skills were more than adequate, I felt I had something to say
but was struggling to sufficiently express myself visually. It was
actually my art tutor who finally pointed out that I might be
working in the wrong medium and suggested I try writing instead. Since that time, I have mainly worked with the written
word but now, inspired by the artistic patient in the chemotherapy suite, I prop myself up in bed with a sketchpad and
my old watercolour set.

I've no fixed idea about what I'm going to paint. I'm not
inspired to capture anything in the room around me, so I
allow my imagination free rein – and the place it takes me
to is the encounters I have experienced with Jesus in prayer.

Falteringly, I begin to paint my inner landscapes. An image of Christ smiling down on a childlike figure tightly curled like a ball. Two silhouettes walking along a wide-open shoreline, past ragged rockpools towards a narrow estuary, a high rock rising in the distance. A flailing figure drawn out by the tide, the descent through the waters, pale light filtering down through the darkness illuminating pale limbs on the seabed. Then a hand reaching down, breaking through the shadowed depths, lifting the broken figure from the ocean floor and raising it up into the light until, finally, two figures stand side by side on that high rock, looking out over the brilliance of the cobalt-blue waters and the pale sands of the land below.

I'm astounded at how easily the images rise again in my mind's eye and, as I paint, I become totally lost in the experience. No sound or thought distracts me as I focus on the simple experience of focusing on Jesus, allowing him to guide my hand. It's as if I am taking something that lies very deep inside me and bringing it out into the light, and I'm utterly absorbed in the process. I was once told by an artist friend of mine that painting is a form of meditation; for a short while, you park your ego and allow the intuitive part of you free rein. It's an idea that the surrealists took to heart in a secular way, seeing painting as a way to tap into one's subconscious, bringing forth images from the depths.

There is, of course, an age-old connection between the visual arts and contemplative prayer, and throughout the centuries art has been one of the key ways that the church has enabled the populace to connect with the divine. Up until the 1450s when the printing press made Scripture available to the masses, it was mainly through paintings, tapestries, sculptures, stained glass and other visual arts that people were able to connect with the Christian narrative, as a majority of people in western Europe were not literate until the seventeenth and eighteenth centuries. And within the church there is also a long tradition of *Visio Divina*, the meaning of which is 'divine seeing' – literally seeing God through the medium of art. Whereas with *Lectio Divina* Scripture is the focal point for meditation, in *Visio Divina* attention is focused onto a work of art, usually of a religious subject. The idea is to begin your contemplation by slowly taking in the colours, shapes and details of a painting, seeing if your attention is drawn to any specific part of the image, and considering what this might be telling you. Then you are invited to respond by praying to God about what has been revealed to you, listening for what he may have to say, and finally to enter that space of deep and silent dwelling in the presence of God.

In addition, there's also a long tradition of praying through the practice of painting which has its roots in the ancient art of iconography, a meditative, prayerful and ritualized art form, in which the materials and the processes as well as the final image have symbolic meaning. The creation of such an icon is seen as a spiritually charged form of meditative prayer, the aim of the icon painter being to create an image that depicts the true inner likeness of Jesus Christ, Mary or one of the saints, and in the Eastern Orthodox Church the icon itself is thought to be imbued with the divine nature of its subject. The actor, musician and convert to Eastern Orthodoxy, Jonathan Jackson, writes of the mystery of art as 'a form of transcendent communication . . . reaching out from the depths of one's soul to engross the imagination and will of another . . . The artist moves by the Spirit and with the Spirit.'[1]

Of course, many Spirit-filled people turn to the visual arts to express a spirituality that goes beyond words, and painting prayer is not limited to the professionals. In fact, perhaps the most wonderful thing about art is that it is accessible to anyone of any age – and the results don't even have to be particularly good. In fact, as I review my creations, I realize that my skills have atrophied over the years through lack of use. They are certainly not great art works but they do express something of my extraordinary encounters with the divine. I won't be showing my paintings to anyone but realize that, in their creation, I have once again connected with something ancient and transcendent.

27

Travelling

As the summer comes to an end, we take a trip to the edge of the North Sea in our camper van. As we drive north, I lie in the back curled up under a blanket, lulled into a half-sleep by the rhythm of wheels on tarmac, enjoying the sensation of being in motion and once again moving towards a new destination.

After a few hours, John wakes me and together we walk a short distance up onto the Yorkshire moors. I can see the strain etched into his face and thank the Lord for this break which is important for both of us. He desperately needs to regain a sense of normality and, as we are nomadic souls, travelling helps to restore our equilibrium. The sun is shining and the purple and gold heather stretches out to the horizon like a lavender seascape. I walk unsteadily up to an elevated point and throw back my head, stretch out my arms and breathe in the late-summer fragrance. Turning on the spot, I am heady with the sense of freedom.

Arriving a few hours later at our destination on the coast, we park up by the sea and John strides out towards the waves carrying his board, the archetypal image of the Australian surfer. It is wonderful to see. I stand on the shoreline, watching his progress, and breathe in the salt-speckled air. I too feel as if I'm in my element.

There's something about the sea that draws humans in at a soul-deep level. Many artists, poets and dreamers have felt its call since time began and, in answer, they find their paths leading to the shoreline; to the edge of the known – and sometimes beyond. Standing on the sandy, rocky outer limits of solid land, we are faced with a seemingly endless horizon, the roaring deep curving away from us as it follows the contours of the earth; the point where the sky touches down upon the sea seemingly full of endless possibility and questions. On the seashore we gaze on eternity, humbled by the mighty force of the ocean. Perhaps what calls us is an innate knowledge that beyond the horizon, beneath the surface of reality, lies a truth stranger and more wonderful than we can imagine. Standing on the shore, caught up in the rhythmic sighing of the sea, it's as if I can hear creation breathing, inhaling and exhaling.

There are only a few other walkers and dogs on the beach, so I comb the shoreline, the tide offering up treasures on the sand: a feather, a skein of seaweed, glistening and green, pebbles shiny and black like jet. I desperately want to be out on the water, but paddleboarding and swimming are still not allowed due to my lack of immunity. So, instead, I remove my trainers and immerse my feet in the shallows, rooting myself in water for a short while at least. As I stand there, the white crests breaking over my feet, I thank the Lord that he has brought me to this place, for the joy of simply being alive this day.

As I walk the dividing line between earth and sea, I watch my feet transformed into something distant, pale and strange by the prism of water. Lulled by the meditative pull of the tide, I lose track of time and, when I look up, I'm surprised how far I have come. Recently I've found it hard to walk even a few hundred yards but I must have wandered for at least a mile or more with my feet in the surf. As I walk back through shallow waters, I have a distinct sense of déjà vu and, when I look around, realize how similar this beach is to the one that I walked with Jesus in my mind's eye – the shoreline I'd recently painted – where he had reassured me that, 'When you pass through the waters, I will be with you' (Isaiah 43:2). It's as if a dream has just broken through into my waking life.

On our return home, the pace picks up and I'm immersed in a round of pre-operative assessments, echocardiograms and blood tests. My nurse equips me with a 'softie', a foam-filled simulation of a breast, and I am encouraged to buy a post-surgery mastectomy bra. In the changing rooms in the department store, I catch sight of my bare torso in the unforgiving full-length mirror. I hardly recognize this swollen, bruised and battered creature and I'm hit by a wave of nostalgia for my pre-cancer self. I realize that, while the bruises from IV lines will fade and the effects of steroids and chemotherapy will wear off, when all this is over, I will be altered irrevocably.

With just twelve days to go until the surgery, my sister picks me up and takes me to her house in Anglesey for one last breath of sea air. We drive across the country and into Wales and, as we wind our way towards the Menai Strait, it's as if I'm travelling back into my past. We both have Celtic souls and there is something about Wales that continues to speak to us both at a very deep level. On the first day we head to Menai Bridge and walk along the Belgian Promenade, breathing in the heady aroma of seaweed and water, the gulls wheeling majestically overhead. We drive the spectacularly winding tree-lined road to Beaumaris and sit beneath the castle walls drinking coffee, eating toasted teacakes and laughing about Bill Bryson's bewilderment at British affection for this humble teatime treat.

We walk along the promenade where once as a student I ate fish and chips on a weekend trip from Aberystwyth and, on the pier, gaze out over the cloud-covered hills of Snowdonia, the high tide chopping at the piles that hold us aloft beneath a fluttering Welsh dragon. The chemotherapy ward and corridors seem a million miles away and, at that moment, I feel as if I've been set free from the fetters of cancer. My imagination wheels overhead above the grey-green waves and the hooded hilltops and on out to sea.

On the second day we drive to the furthest reaches of the island, to the shore at Rhosneigr. The autumn chill is drawing in, but my sister, an enthusiastic advocate of cold-water therapy, is determined to swim in the sea. I sit on the sand and, as Charlotte purposefully strides towards the water, watch the landscape unfolding in layers of colour: the pale gold of the dry sand, the silvery grey of the Irish Sea, interspersed with islands of ochre rock forced up from the depths of the earth over millennia. Beyond the sea line rises the mottled late-afternoon sky, shades of pink bleeding through the darkening clouds. Nearby, a child kicks at the sand, joined in his unbridled enthusiasm by a mud-splattered Jack Russell. Out at sea my sister's head bobs up and down between the waves like a shoreline seal. I feel so utterly alive in the open air with the endless horizon stretching out before me. I pick up handfuls of perfectly formed cockle shells and put them in my pocket as a reminder of this glorious moment.

Back at home, I prepare myself for the forthcoming surgery. A couple of days before I'm scheduled to go to the hospital, I join the Encounter group for a prayer session. As I close my eyes and follow the prompting of the facilitator, I once again see Jesus in my mind's eye. I know it is Jesus but

I cannot make out the details of his face. This is not the version of Christ who walked with me along the seashore of my mind. The presence that I now encounter seems less human; he is both embodied and disembodied.

I imagine that I am lying prone on an operating table as he stands beside me but also flows all around me. Then, in my mind's eye, he bends down, puts his hands on my torso and opens me up, exposing my muscles, nerves and veins in all their gory glory. It's a truly disturbing mental image which becomes even more macabre as he climbs up onto the table and reaches into the gaping wound in the centre of my body, gradually moving within me, becoming one with me until he fills every part of my body. Now his face occupies my face, his mouth becomes mine and, as he fills every fibre of my body, there's no space left for the cancer. He is flowing in around me, extending far beyond into the eternity of the universe, and through and into my very being. As I lie there on the operating table of my mind, the words of John's gospel come to me: 'Abide in me, and I in you' (John 15:4 KJV). *Christ above me, Christ below me, Christ within me.*

The day before the surgery, I'm scheduled to attend a different hospital to have an injection of a radioactive tracer. At the same time as the mastectomy, the surgeon plans to perform a sentinel node biopsy (the removal of the main lymph node under my right arm) in order to determine whether the cancer has once again spread to my lymph system. This is a completely new experience, as the last time I had cancer it was patently obvious that the cancer had metastasized. This time, however, the scans have indicated that there may be an issue but are not conclusive.

The day before the planned procedure, I go online to find out more about what is involved and am horrified to read that, twenty-four hours before the surgery, tracer material is injected into the nipple area! A prospect that I find profoundly disturbing. So far, I have not been overly worried about the surgery itself, but overnight I wind myself up as tight as a spring about this injection. So much so that by the time I arrive at the hospital I feel nauseous.

I lie down on the reclining chair, close my eyes and clutch my cross, saying a silent prayer for strength, and wait for the onset of searing pain. Only to hear the nurse say: 'All done; you can get dressed again now.'

'What? I didn't feel anything!'

'No, it's a tiny needle – very few people do.'

I feel such a fool and, as I explain to her how wound up I have been, I laugh so much that I nearly cry and, as I walk out of the hospital again, I recognize that the laughter has broken the in-evitable pre-operative tension. As I head home, I feel lighter and calmer and the surgery no longer feels like such a major under-taking. God is on the case and the NHS perform over eighteen thousand mastectomies a year, so I have nothing to fear.

On the day of the surgery, I wake before dawn and say the Daily Office and listen to *The Bible in One Year*. The psalm for the day is 103, the scripture that has followed me through-out both cancer journeys and is such an expression of assur-ance in God's healing:

Praise the LORD, O my soul,
>   all my inmost being, praise his holy name . . .
> who . . . heals all your diseases,
> who redeems your life from the pit . . .

vv. 1–4

The words once again feel like a benediction.

To avoid the risk of Covid at the main site, the surgeon is going to operate on me at a nearby private hospital which has been co-opted for the day. I am the first on the list, so we arrive just before eight o'clock in the morning. John isn't allowed to accompany me, so we sit together in the car and pray before he leaves me at the door.

I'm immediately struck by how different the private hospital environment is from an NHS hospital. Once beyond the plush reception, it's evident that the hospital is only geared up for day surgery. I'm shown to a minuscule cubicle rather like those at swimming pools, equipped with a plastic chair and a locker, and am soon joined by an alarming number of medics – a nurse with a clipboard, the surgeon, an anaesthetist and one other doctor – who squeeze themselves into the cubicle alongside me. We are crammed together like sardines in a can and I try to keep a straight face as the surgeon shifts everyone around so that she can draw a number of large circles on the right side of my chest with a black felt-tip pen. As I change into a hospital gown, I steal one last look at my graffitied torso and say goodbye to my right breast. It has served me well, but I no longer have any qualms about its departure. I know it's for the best.

Dressed in a blue paper gown, pink paper hat and mask, I'm escorted down the corridor and into the operating theatre. Over the years I've had numerous operations, but it's the first time that I have arrived at the theatre on my own two feet and without the benefit of pre-medication and I find it a surreal experience to be fully alert in this unfamiliar environment. I climb onto the narrow operating table and, as the team around me busy themselves with preparations, I look around and observe the paraphernalia of medical intervention: a trolley laid out with various surgical instruments that would not look out of place in a torture chamber and, above my head, a vast manoeuvrable lighting system. In addition to the surgeon whom I already know, there is a second medic who is dressed in a hijab. She stands by me and speaks calming words in a gentle voice.

The anaesthetist initially fails to find a vein into which to insert a cannula, but brings out an ultrasound machine and, to my relief, a vein is found and a line is inserted. An oxygen mask is placed over my face and the room begins to recede. In my hand, I can just feel the contours of my wooden cross.

Coming to in a recovery room is always a disorienting experience. It's like being yanked suddenly and reluctantly out of a deliciously deep sleep, only to find that someone is stabbing your body with sharp knives. Someone in my peripheral vision offers me pain relief and, as the pain begins to recede, I look down and register that one side of my body is flat. It feels slightly surreal but there is no revulsion, only a sense of utter relief.

On my right side, a slightly macabre bottle of what looks like blood is attached to my body by a tube; this is the wound drain, the aspect I hated most about my previous cancer surgery, but it's an essential part of the healing process. My wooden cross lies on the blanket. I imagine it must have fallen from my hand as I went under, and I'm grateful that someone rescued it and reunited us.

The surgeon materializes at my side, and reassures me that all went smoothly.

I mumble my gratitude.

She tells me, 'We've taken the sentinel node and we will have the results in two weeks' time. Then we'll know if we need further surgery.'

I try not to think about this prospect and just take today as a win. I drift back into half-sleep.

After a while, I feel more alert and am wheeled back and installed in what appears to be a dentist's chair. Now that I am sitting up, I'm given a cup of tea and two small packets of custard creams. I can't remember anything tasting quite so good. I demolish the biscuits while messaging my darling John and the kids. A text comes back from my youngest asking, 'Can I call you the one-tit wonder?' I laugh until it hurts. I think I'm on a post-operative adrenalin high.

I post a picture on my Facebook page of myself – bald, grinning, buoyed by biscuits and excess adrenalin – and I enjoy reading the various messages, which are variously hilarious and spiritual:

'That's great news!!! But custard creams??? Surely worth a chocolate hobnob?'

'Hey – you are in the one-tit gang now (at least until your next operation).'

'Thanks be to God. Hallelujah. May you have swift healing.'

Time passes remarkably quickly. By two o'clock in the afternoon, I'm judged well enough to be sent home and, before being discharged, I'm given an impressive array of painkillers and a floral handbag in which to carry the bottle from my wound drain. Back in the cubicle, I take a peek at the scar as I change back into my clothes. It's very neat and I say to myself, *Yes, I am okay with this.* Somehow the idea of being mutilated has turned out to be much worse than the reality.

Then, just six hours after arriving for surgery, I totter rather unsteadily out of the hospital and into the arms of my husband.

28

Aftermath

Once I'm home I settle back into the bosom of my family, wrapped in a comfortable haze of anaesthetic. In some ways, it's a relief to be in my own home but, at the same time, it does feel strange to be ejected from the reassurance of the hospital so quickly. In the 'old days' mastectomy patients would automatically be admitted to hospital for at least an overnight stay, but contemporary thinking is that healing takes place more rapidly in a familiar environment.

As the afternoon wears on, however, I become conscious of a pain in my right calf. Having spent so much of my life on long-haul flights, I'm acutely alert to the danger of deep vein thrombosis (DVT), particularly as there is a history of DVTs in my family. I tell myself it's very unlikely that a problem would develop so soon after surgery but, as the evening wears on, the pain becomes worse and my calf begins to throb.

The later it gets, the more alert I begin to feel. Perhaps it's the anaesthesia wearing off, or the copious amount of tea I consumed immediately post-surgery, but sleep is elusive. At around one o'clock in the morning, I read the post-operative literature I was given on my way out and realize that there may in fact be a problem which I should not leave until morning. I ring the private hospital line but there is no answer. So, I ring the only out-of-hours number I know – that of the acute oncology line – and they give me the usual advice. So, at two o'clock in the morning, John takes me yet again to the A&E department.

The unit is heaving and as I join the masses – which include a very vocal drunk who's weaving his way around between the other patients – the irony is not lost on me that the risk of catching Covid is considerably higher in A&E than if I'd been kept on a ward overnight. John checks me in, explaining that I've had surgery that morning, and I'm seen almost immediately by a young triage nurse who examines my leg and then disappears in search of an emergency doctor.

A few minutes later she returns armed with a syringe of a blood thinner called dalteparin. It's too late to have a doppler scan which will determine whether I do actually have a blood clot, and there is quite a waiting list, so for safety's sake the doctor has recommended that I am given a box of syringes which I'm to inject into my abdomen on a daily basis. I'm there for a grand total of just forty minutes, which has to be a record turnaround for an overstretched A&E department, and by three o'clock in the morning we are heading home on empty roads.

The following morning, I feel surprisingly well but, as the day progresses, and the last effects of the anaesthetic wear off, I have to break open the painkillers. The first one I try makes me so dizzy that I need to lie down again, and I decide I would rather deal with the pain. In the afternoon, a nurse phones to check in on me and tells me off for not wearing my post-surgery bra and 'softie', which apparently helps with the healing, so when I come off the phone I enlist John's help to insert me into the contraption. I'd never intended for John to see the wound (I'd rather unrealistically planned to keep the top part of my body covered at all times from now on), but in my current state there is no alternative. As he approaches the task, he is completely unfazed, although as he is not particularly adept at dealing with women's lingerie I end up with one side considerably higher than the other, which provides some comic relief.

Early in the evening, my youngest emerges from her room and, sitting down beside me, looks alarmed. 'Mum, there's blood on your pyjamas!'

I look down and sure enough there is a large patch of blood on the new silk pyjamas I had rather impractically bought for the occasion.

'Oh God, Mum's bleeding out!'

John comes over and checks on me. By this time, my child is scaling the heights of teenage anxiety, crying 'Oh my God, are you going to die?'

I try to calm her down and tell her that, of course, I'm not going to die: 'It's only a bit of blood, and that's quite normal after an operation.' However, I agree to ring the hospital if it will reassure her.

I call the private hospital number but am quickly rebuffed by a nurse who tells me that their responsibility ended with the surgery. Her only advice is that I go back to A&E, a prospect I just can't face, so I call my local GP surgery and manage to speak to the duty doctor just before she leaves. 'You're home already?' she asks in apparent amazement. 'Pre-Covid you would have been there three or four days!' She adds, 'I wouldn't worry about the blood, though.' I share the doctor's assurances with my panicking child and peace is restored.

However, when I wake the following morning, there's a significant amount of blood on the bedsheets. Once again, I ring the hospital and am assured that this is perfectly normal. A nurse tells me that the wound for the drain isn't sealed, so some bleeding is to be expected. I try to get up and keep mobile but, as the day progresses, I start to feel increasingly weak and dizzy. By early afternoon, I no longer feel strong enough to sit up, so go back to bed where I drift in and out of sleep for the remainder of the day.

The following morning, the third after the operation, I wake with the dawn but am so weak I can barely lift my head off the pillow. Once again, I lie in bed, drifting and listening to *The Bible in One Year* passages and commentary for the day which make the point that the Lord can be glorified in defeat.[1] The psalm for the day is 118 and the familiar words:

> I will not die but live,
>   and will proclaim what the LORD has done.
>
> v. 17

When I finally try to rise, the room spins around me like a carousel and, as I place my feet on the floor, the ground seems to move away beneath me. Looking down I notice that the whole of the right side of my body and the bedsheets are covered in blood and, for the first time, I feel a sense of genuine alarm. Something isn't right here. Fumbling, I pick up the mobile on my bedside table and ring the hospital again. This time I speak to a different, but equally patient, nurse who tells me that this is all completely normal, and that the intense dizziness is a response to the anaesthetic that's still in my system, and that the blood will be leakage from the drain wound.

This time, however, I don't feel the same sense of reassurance. I sit on the side of the bed, the windows and doors shifting around me, pondering what I've been told. I know many others who have been through this surgery and none of them ever mentioned a subsequent bloodbath, and surely the effects of the anaesthetic should be wearing off by now, not getting progressively worse? I tell myself that thousands of women have this procedure done very year; that it is considered minor enough surgery to be treated as a day case. Surely the nurses would know if there was something wrong, but somewhere in my subconscious an alarm bell is ringing.

That afternoon, I'm due to go for the long overdue doppler scan of my leg to ascertain if I do actually have a DVT (although the dalteparin I've been faithfully injecting myself with every day is likely to have already dissolved any clots that might have been there). John comes upstairs and helps me with the disarmingly difficult task of getting dressed, and holds my limp body under the shoulders as I try to negotiate the stairs. When he plants me on the sofa, I'm unable to sit upright and slump like a rag doll that has lost its stuffing.

'It's okay,' I tell him. 'We'll be at the hospital in a couple of hours for the scan – they can have a look at me then.'

John, who has so far been remarkably sanguine, now looks genuinely alarmed and, as more blood begins to seep through my shirt, he bites the bullet and calls an ambulance.

For me, the siren of an ambulance has always had a ring of finality about it. I was the one who called the ambulance for my father on his last day and for my mother when she left her beloved home for the last time. In Corfu, it was my sister and I who called the local ambulance and helped the Greek paramedics take my aunt down the narrow stairs from her garret flat just before she died.

Now the fact that my husband, whose default position on illnesses tends to be Pollyanna-like denial, has resorted to calling an ambulance fills me with a strange mixture of calm and foreboding. I don't feel anxious or afraid but rather like a cinema-goer who has worked out the ending of the film and is now simply watching events spiral towards their inevitable conclusion.

The action seems to take place in slow motion. At first, I see a flash of black and white in my peripheral vision and then the living room seems to fill to the brim with the presence of paramedics. One takes my blood pressure and my oxygen saturation, while another examines the doorways.

The older paramedic then kneels down beside the sofa, his face close enough for me to see his wrinkles, and says quietly, but deliberately, 'I'm going to be honest with you. I can't tell you this is going to be hunky-dory. I think it's likely that you have a pulmonary embolism and we need to get you to hospital right now.'

I nod compliantly and they spring into action. The large wooden coffee table in the centre of the room is pushed to one side, the French doors are thrown open, the haze of jasmine that surrounds the door is parted, and a trolley lifted in. The whole scene seems incongruous.

John hovers, stricken, holding my hand as they scoop me off the sofa and place my bloody body on the crisp white sheets. I no longer have the strength to move or speak. Utterly passive, I watch the events unfold with a sense of curious detachment. As I'm carried out of the French windows and through the garden, it feels surreal to be watching my home recede from view from this unfamiliar angle. I thank the Lord that my youngest is at school and that my eldest isn't home to witness my departure.

As I'm lifted into the ambulance, John stands in the road, bereft and helpless. The paramedic asks if he wants to come and say goodbye to me. He nods mutely and climbs into the ambulance.

'I'm afraid you can't go with her, mate. Covid restrictions.'

'Can I follow in my car?'

'Sorry, mate, they won't let you in.'

A bear of a man, he towers over me, my protector, my sanctuary, my soulmate. My voice sounds unfamiliar as I tell him, 'I love you so much.'

He nods, his face bathed in tears. 'I love you too.'

After nearly thirty years of laughter, tears, discoveries and losses, when it comes to it there are no other words.

He climbs down out of the ambulance and, as the door closes on my love, I catch one last glimpse of him standing in the road, silently weeping.

29

Destination

As we leave the village and bounce and wind our way along the narrow country roads, the male paramedic sits with me, watching the blood pressure monitor. I hear the driver phone through to the local hospital telling them that they 'have a PE coming in'.

Inside the ambulance the pain intensifies. Perhaps it's the movement; ambulances are not the most comfortable of rides even if you're not the one on the trolley. I'm not afraid. Instead, I have a sense of detached curiosity. The inside of the vehicle looks rather like the interior of a space module, the walls lined with metal cabinets full of equipment, locked away in case they float off through lack of gravity. The paramedic keeps up a cheerful banter, no doubt to distract me, but all I really want is quiet.

When we reach the hospital, I'm unloaded like a parcel and pushed down pale-lemon corridors. Strip lights flash by above me like road markings, until I'm reversed into a bay, with a blue privacy curtain drawn around. Having delivered me, the paramedics melt away and I'm finally left alone.

I'm too tired to be scared. I close my eyes and begin to drift. Once again, I am at sea, lulled by the seeming movement of the water, too exhausted to fight the inevitable descent, and as the tide takes me I surrender and slide further from the light.

A pressure on my arm drags me back to the surface. I open my eyes to find two doctors standing over me, one of whom is taking my blood pressure. He reads off the numbers blinking on a portable digital screen.

'Fifty over thirty, heart rate dropped'.

Even in my passive state, I register that this isn't good. Then all hell breaks loose.

The doctor shouts 'Resusc!' and the cry echoes through the bays, repeated and passed on like a Chinese whisper.

I'm struggling to stay awake.

Then, once again I am in motion, surrounded by a sea of cyan scrubs. Behind the sea of faces, lights recede at alarming speed.

I float, substance suspended.

I'm now in a very small room surrounded by a large number of fast-moving medics. I am at the centre of a hurricane of activity but, in the eye of the storm, all is still. While medics bark orders, I am tranquil.

'Catherine, Catherine. Can you hear us?'

Who's Catherine?

'Catherine, we need to give you four units of blood very fast. Your heart may not be able to cope with being given that much blood at once, but if we don't your heart is going to stop anyway.'

'CATHERINE. Do you give permission?'

I wave my hand in a vague gesture of royal assent and mumble 'A-negative'.

'Who's your next of kin?'

I think of John. *Poor John. My darling John.* A junior doctor holds up a small black duffel bag, that was hurriedly packed, and rummaging through it pulls out my phone.

Someone must have accessed the emergency number because I realize that the medic beside me is talking to my husband. *Oh, my darling John.*

I become momentarily conscious of a searing pain in my arm and realize that someone is trying to insert a cannula. Through the haze, I catch the word 'theatre'.

An urgent thought surfaces. *My cross, I must have my cross.* I gesticulate towards the doctor, who is still holding my black bag, and try to vocalize the words 'My cross'. The clamour around me is so loud that I'm unsure if she can hear me, but she rifles through the bag and holds up my wooden clutch cross.

She places the cross in my left hand and folds my arm over the surface of the blanket. I close my eyes and sink back into the comfort of the waters.

Suddenly the seabed seems to shift beneath me and once again I am flashing down corridors, propelled by blue-clothed attendants.

I ask the air 'What's happening?'

A tall bespectacled figure who appears to be running beside my head replies, 'This is one of those very rare complications that we really don't want to happen after surgery. We're going to the theatre.'

'What about my lungs?' I ask plaintively.

'We need to save your life first!'

He peels away as we turn into the operating theatre and a familiar face looms in over me – the female Muslim medic who had been in the operating theatre during my mastectomy. She smiles over me kindly.

I realize that someone is trying to get a cannula into my hand again but I now feel utterly detached. There is no more pain, just a creeping sensation that makes its way up my right

arm, and I begin to fade. The bespectacled face of the anaesthetist hovers over me, oxygen mask in hand, and the stark
realization that has been hovering in the wings comes centre
stage: *I may not wake up from this procedure.*

There is no panic, only a recognition that this is where my
journey has been leading to all along.

As the mask descends and my eyes close, the faces of those
I have loved so dearly pass before me.

My darling John, the love of my life.

My beautiful eldest child, so strong and independent. My
beloved first child.

My youngest, so brave, always marching to the beat of her
own drum, and so precious.

My sister, Charlotte, full of wisdom and comfort.

One by one, I try to convey to them, wordlessly, the enormity of my love.

Then, as I begin to slip into unconsciousness, something
ancient, wonderful and unfathomable begins to rise up from
the oceanic depths of my being.

An indescribable power ascending from the shadowy
depths,
surging up through the waters of my soul
until it breaks through the surface.
Consuming me,
inhabiting every fibre of my being.
And in the final moment of awareness,
there is but a single thought . . .
Jesus.

Epilogue

It was only two days later that I became fully aware of how close I had come to death. At which point I was told that I had suffered a major internal haemorrhage and a peri-arrest of the heart due to a massive loss of blood.

I had been kept alive long enough to be operated on by a series of blood transfusions, but my life had continued to hang in the balance for another twenty-four hours as the doctors walked a very fine line, administering more blood thinners to counter what appeared to be multiple potentially fatal blood clots in my lungs, while at the same time trying not to induce another haemorrhage.

While I was in the operating theatre, my poor family had been to hell and back as they sat waiting for the phone to ring and for someone to tell them whether I was alive or dead. My heart aches when I think about what they went through.

There are two very important points that I must make. First of all, my experience of chemotherapy side effects was fairly extreme and most people will find cancer treatments far easier to handle than I did. Second, if you are facing a potential mastectomy, please do *not* be put off by what happened to me. My experience is incredibly rare (which is probably why the seriousness of my situation was not initially apparent) and

the wonderful NHS surgeons perform thousands of successful and uneventful mastectomies every year. Overall, I cannot
praise staff at all levels highly enough for their compassion,
professionalism and perseverance. The surgeons and staff who
attended me on that fateful day undoubtedly saved my life.

The original surgery was a success; the sentinel node biopsy mercifully came back as negative and all traces of cancer
were removed by the mastectomy. After six weeks' recovery
from the following emergency surgery, I was also successfully
treated with radiotherapy and monoclonal antibody treatments and I am now in full remission. I've now started on a
five-year course of the hormone treatment exemestane, and
such is my confidence in the NHS that I will soon be going
under the knife again to have the second mastectomy. I don't
believe that the attending staff could have done any more for
me, and I will be profoundly grateful to them for the rest of
my days, however many they may be.

Despite the medical complications and dramas – or perhaps because of them – this has been an extraordinary time
of discovery that began with my sepsis-induced ocean floor
experience and reached its zenith in those final moments of
consciousness as I hovered between life and death on the operating table. Cancer became for me a gateway into a different
and more intuitive connection with my Creator, a relationship
nurtured through spiritual disciplines that hark back to the
very origins of Christianity. It is not easy to write about an
apophatic experience, but I hope that I have conveyed something of the poignancy and power of those experiences which
changed the way that I understand and approach the world
and God.

It was only when I had nearly finished writing this book that I recalled an incident, recorded in my memoir *Sea Changed*, that had a profound impact on my life and faith. I was 29 years old and was staying in a beach hut on the Thai island of Koh Samet alongside another group of travellers. Every morning I would walk down the pristine beach and swim out into perfect pale-azure waters. I felt perfectly safe, but one morning I swam out too far and, lulled by the silence out at sea, I didn't notice the wind that had begun to whip across the surface. I soon found I could only catch glimpses of the beach through the peaks and troughs of water.

I tried to swim back towards shore but found that I had to fight to keep afloat and, as I breathed deeply, salt water stung my throat. I eventually began to tire and the waves broke over my head until, aching, I began to sink down through the pale-blue water. Above my head I could see the churning waves, but below I drifted in silence. My chest ached but my eyes were clear as I gazed around me. I sank further down and let the waters enfold me. All was still. A profound sense of peace came over me. I recognized that I was drowning but felt an inexplicable sense of calm and, as I sank down beneath the waves, I had the impression of being comforted, of being held. In the depths of the water, I had a powerful sense that I was not alone, and that I was utterly loved.

I was rescued by one of my fellow travellers who heroically swam out, dived down, and dragged me back up into the air and back to shore, where I lay choking, vomiting, and heaving pain-filled gasps of air. For this, I am still deeply grateful but, in the months afterwards, I was unable to shake the conviction that, down in the depths, I had encountered something profound, mysterious and divine. As I recovered, I was struck by a profound sense of nostalgia, a bittersweet yearning for that sense of being held – of being wrapped in love – that had come to me as I sank beneath the waves.

It was only as I finished the first draft of this book that I made this connection, which is remarkable given that my near-drowning off the coast of Thailand was, in fact, a pivotal moment in my faith journey and a first step on the path back to Christ. Although I didn't realize it at the time, water flows through the pages of the Bible and is symbolic of the Spirit of God. Jesus described himself as the source of this 'living water', saying: "'If anyone is thirsty, let him come to me and drink. Whoever believes in me, as the Scripture has said, streams of living water will flow within him." By this he meant the Spirit' (John 7:37–39). He is the water that flows around us and within us, the Spirit from whom we cannot be separated by suffering or pain. For:

> Where can I go from your Spirit?
>> Where can I flee from your presence?
> If I go up to the heavens, you are there;
>> if I make my bed in the depths, you are there.
>
> Psalm 139:7–8

I now also see that my 'ocean floor' experience in that hospital room was the starting point of a new and extraordinary journey that, over the course of my treatment, took me even deeper into the mystery of a God whose nature cannot be contained by our imagination or language, but who made his love and power known to me when I most needed him.

I don't know if my ocean floor experience in the midst of cancer was a vision, the result of delirium, or a waking dream, but I can see some parallels with the experiences of Christian mystics, ancient and modern. Certainly, some aspects of this journey have been hard to understand, let alone explain, but the whole of Christian faith requires us to accept a mystery that our human minds cannot really comprehend: a deity who alone is the source of all reality, the Creator who set the spark that ignited the universe into being, but who is also three in one. God the Father, Son and Holy Spirit – three but of one essence. He is also the God who both transcends our reality and has fully inhabited our existence, walking the earth incarnate in a human frame. Who broke the bounds of death and now continues to exist not only in that dimension known as heaven but also within humanity itself in the form of the Holy Spirit. It is incomprehensible, but didn't God himself say:

> My thoughts are not your thoughts,
> > neither are your ways my ways . . .
> As the heavens are higher than the earth,
> > so are my ways higher than your ways
> > and my thoughts than your thoughts.

> Isaiah 55:8–9

In my book *Soul's Scribe*, I explored what the Franciscan friar Richard Rohr has described as a second-half-of-life faith in which, on the precipice of understanding, we experience a surrender of our intellectual certainty and a humility in the face of the vast mystery of reality. For much of my life, my faith has been head-driven as I have pored over the Bible, the-ological commentaries and the writings of spiritual greats in an attempt to better understand the mystery of God and reconcile the paradoxes of faith. But in the process of facing my own mortality, I now seem to have entered this different stage of faith, in which I am more able to surrender the rationalist's need to always 'know' and instead to embrace the mystery that is Yahweh, the Alpha and the Omega, the beginning and the end of things. As I look back over this experience, I am able to pray, like the psalmist, 'Such knowledge is too wonderful for me, too lofty for me to attain' (Psalm 139:6); to place my trust in the greater Healer and to pray 'Thy will be done' and truly mean it.

Jung believed that the purpose of understanding one's personality profile was not to justify one's actions and approach to life, but rather to identify the opposite of our natural tendencies and to learn to grow into this. And I can now see that God has been leading me on this journey of development; from a judger's need to control to a greater willingness to embrace the ambiguity of unknowing, and the ability to *qavah*: to wait in anticipation and 'live the situation out to the full in the belief that something hidden there will manifest itself to us.'[1] Through my enforced isolation he has also nurtured and grown the introverted part of my personality, leading me into a new kind of relationship with him, opening up an intuitive connection at the deepest levels of my consciousness. A connection with the God in whom we live and move and have our being but who also dwells within us; a connection first felt during suffering and rekindled through the spiritual discipline of meditation.

It is, however, a journey that has only just begun. As I return to life, I also realize that my experience in the depths has changed the way that I view the world; that I am more able to see Christ in those around me. It's as if, having broken back out into the daylight, I see with new eyes the glimpses of the kingdom all around us, and, the more time I spend in the depths, the clearer that vision becomes.

I no longer use the mantra like a hammer to batter down the thoughts that distract, but have learned to sit with God in the stillness of my soul, to simply *be*. I have also replaced the mantra *Ma-ra-na-tha* with the sacred word that came to me when I stood on the border between life and death: Jesus. That simple name, above every other, that encompasses not only the unimaginable majesty and power of the being that existed before time and space and spoke the universe into being but also the incomprehensible beauty of God-incarnate who walked among us and suffered all the pain and grief that can be inflicted on humankind, suffering his own 'dark night of the soul' before eventually giving up his life. Jesus the source of life in whom we abide and who abides within us. If there is a word that can encompass the being who created everything in existence, who pervades every atom of the universe, and who is love, the dynamic force that brought us to life; if there are syllables that can signify the force in which we live and move and have our being, and who lives within the very depths of our souls, then it has to be quite simply – *Jesus*.

I cannot bear to think about the fact that I so nearly left my family in such a shocking manner, but what I do know is that if I had died on that operating table then I would still have been healed at a very fundamental level. What rose up from within me unbidden that day was love beyond imagining, a love that surrounds and fills us, enables us to see through God's eyes those around us and to appreciate how much they too are loved. It's a love that overflows from our being into the world around us, touching those we encounter, and that love has a name. It's Jesus, the Christ in whom we live and move and have our being, who also inexplicably exists within us. It's the God whom I came face to face with on the ocean floor of my own suffering, with whom I have been nurturing my relationship in the stillness and the silence, and who came to me in my moment of greatest need.

At the beginning of this journey I was given the promise that God had plans to give me hope and a future, but there was also a second part to that promise: 'Then you will call upon me and come and pray to me, and I will listen to you. You will seek me and find me when you seek me with all your heart' (Jer. 29:12–13). Like all of us, I don't know for how much longer I will walk this earth, but what I do know is that, on that day when I am finally led beyond the shallows and sink beneath the waves for the last time, he will be there in the depths, waiting for me on the ocean floor.

Afterword

It is my hope and prayer that my journey may encourage you, and inspire you to also explore a more intuitive connection with God through meditation as part of your prayer life. In my case it was the experience of cancer that led me towards a deeper experience of God, but it really isn't necessary to suffer in order to come before the Lord in this way. It also isn't necessary to go into retreat from the world and to isolate oneself; there's a long tradition of contemplative and meditative prayer in the church. In fact, my own diocese, that of Oxford, seeks to be a Christ-like church that is contemplative, compassionate and courageous (and has even created an educational toolkit on contemplative practices for schools which includes a form of breath-based meditation or 'stilling'). Christian meditation is also not a replacement for other forms of prayer, but the spiritual discipline of meditation can be for us a gateway through which we enter into a more intuitive relationship with the Father, bringing us into the presence of the Alpha and Omega and opening up a dialogue of the soul that goes beyond words.

There are many different paths to Christian meditation; no one's journey towards that liminal place will be the same and each of our experiences will be unique. Depending on your personality type, you may think that one type of prayer will come to you more naturally than another. Logic, for example, would tell us that an extrovert soul might be better able to connect with God by vocalizing prayer, either alone or with others, and that an introvert, who is more energized by solitude, might find contemplative prayer a more natural fit. But as someone whom Jung would have undoubtedly classified as an extrovert, and as a writer who has spent her life working with words, I have come to love my time in the stillness with God that goes beyond language. In fact, I can no longer imagine my life without the profound depth of that connection. That doesn't mean that I don't sometimes struggle to quieten the internal chatter of my mind. There are many days when my thoughts seem to be constantly pulling me back to the surface, but the more I meditate, the more often I catch glimpses of deeper waters. The important thing is to persevere.

Meditative prayer should not, however, become a burden. Ancient teachers and modern masters such as John Main say that you should devote twenty to thirty minutes to meditation at the beginning and end of the day. However, it's important to recognize that these teachers were all speaking out of the context of monastic life. For most of us who have jobs, families and other responsibilities, this kind of commitment may seem completely unrealistic and may put you off the idea of exploring Christian meditation. (I own up to the fact that I have managed to meditate both morning and evening a grand total of three times, and during one of my evening meditations I actually fell asleep!) The important thing is to just try to carve out some time in your day when you can make the space to seek God in silence and stillness. This can be in the morning or evening, or perhaps another time of day when you can 'go into your room, close the door and pray to your Father, who is unseen' (Matthew 6:6). It can be helpful to have a particular place to meditate, but that space can be anywhere where you can find stillness (I often walk up the fields above our village to Cowper's Alcove to meditate). Some translations speak of an 'inner room' and I like to think of this as any location where you can access your own 'inner room' – that place of stillness.

You may also be tempted to wait for the 'right' time to meditate; for a moment of calm in your life. But, as I hope my story has shown, it's perhaps in the midst of the storm that we most need to find that stillness within that enables us to come most fully into God's presence. It was when I was at perhaps the lowest point in my life, when my very life itself was threatened, that I most needed to reach him in the depths. There is great power to prayer in the midst of the storm, and resting in the presence of the Lord can bring a peace that really does pass all understanding. A period of meditation is also time invested in building the foundations of a life filled with love, and in the transformation of the mind that enables us to see others as God sees them, as beloved children of God. It's about opening the eyes of our hearts to the all-surpassing power and love that is God, and allowing that love to overflow into our lives and to touch the lives of those we encounter. In itself, to meditate is to love.

I hope very much that you will be encouraged by my story to take the first steps on a journey into deeper connection with God and, if you would like to know more about how to approach Christian meditation, the following resources may be of interest. This is not a comprehensive list – there are very many teachers and resources available to those who want to explore Christian meditation – but these are the resources that I was blessed with as I explored, and I pray that they may also be a blessing to you.

Resources

Lectio Divina

Lectio 365 is a free app which provides a daily devotional that helps you pray the Bible every day.

Written by leaders from the 24-7 Prayer movement, Lectio 365 provides Scripture and an audio that guides you through the process of *Lectio* with the option of morning and evening meditations.

Christian mindfulness

Introducing Christian Mindfulness by Richard H.H. Johnston (2015) provides a valuable introduction to the principles and practice of Christian mindfulness and is an entry point to his course, which I followed. His website https://christianmind fulness.co.uk has full details of his courses and events, including free introductory videos and mindfulness meditations. Johnston also leads the Mindful Church which at the time of writing meets online on a weekly basis. Johnston also runs a course which covers other types of contemplative prayer, including *Lectio Divina* meditation.

Christian mantra-based meditation

The World Community for Christian Meditation (WCCM) is a global spiritual community of meditators in over 100 countries united by John Main, Benedictine monk and teacher of mantra-based meditation. The WCCM website https://wccm .org/ has a wealth of resources, including introductory videos, online courses, live streams of meditations and services from the WCCM retreat centre, the Bonnevaux Centre for Peace, as well as reflections and information about retreats. You can also download a free app which includes meditation resources, articles and seminars as well as a podcast.

Centering Prayer

Contemplative Outreach is an international and interdenominational community of individuals and small faith communities established by Father Thomas Keating, one of the founders of the Centering Prayer movement – a form of contemplative prayer which involves focus on a single sacred word to still the mind and enable us to come into the presence of God. In Centering Prayer this sacred word is not used throughout, as in the approach proposed by John Main, but rather as a means of refocusing our awareness when our thoughts draw us away from the well of inner stillness. This is the approach that I have now adopted, focusing on the sacred word given to me in my hour of greatest need – Jesus.

Contemplative Outreach's website https://www.contempla tiveoutreach.org/ provides guidance, access to online support groups, courses, retreats and other resources. You can also download Contemplative Outreach's mobile app Centering Prayer on the App Store or the Google Play store. This app helps to lead you into meditation and includes an opening scripture of your choice, a timer and a closing prayer or reflection.

Breast cancer resources

If you want to know more about breast cancer, how to detect the condition and treatments, or access support, I suggest that you go to the Breast Cancer Now website; https://breastcancernow.org is the place to go to find out anything to do with breast cancer and I am so grateful for the support they have given me on both my cancer journeys.

Macmillan are also amazing and I don't know what I would have done without their advice and help during this time. Through their website https://www.macmillan.org.uk you can access a very wide range of practical help, from detailed information about treatments to assistance in dealing with your finances during cancer, as well as their helpline.

Finally, please, please be vigilant and make sure you take up the offer of a mammogram or persuade your loved ones to do the same – it may just save a life.

Bibliography

Anonymous. *The Cloud of Unknowing and Other Works* (trans. A.C. Spearing; London: Penguin Classics, 2001).

Capps, Charles. *God's Creative Power® for Healing* (Broken Arrow, OK: Charles Capps Publishing, 1991).

Common Worship: Services and Prayers for the Church of England (Church House Publishing: The Archbishops Council, 2000).

Curtis, Ken. *Reflections on the Beatitudes for People with Cancer: A Personal Journey Presented by Ken Curtis* (Worcester, PA: Vision Video, 2013).

Dossey MD, Larry. *Healing Words: The Power of Prayer and the Practice of Medicine* (San Francisco, CA: HarperCollins Publishers, 1993).

Freeman, Laurence. *John Main: Essential Writings. Selected with an introduction by Laurence Freeman* (Maryknoll, NY: Orbis Books, 2002).

Griffiths, Bede. *The Marriage of East and West* (Tucson, AZ: Medio Media, 1976).

Herndon, Jaime R. 'The History of Cancer: Discovery and Treatment', *Very Well Health*, 11 Dec. 2022. https://www.verywellhealth.com/the-history-of-cancer-514101 (accessed 14 Feb. 2023).

Jackson, Jonathan. *The Mystery of Art: Becoming an Artist in the Image of God* (Chesterton, IN: Ancient Faith Publishing, 2014).

Johnston, Richard H.H. *Introducing Christian Mindfulness* (self-published, 2015).

Main, John. *Christian Meditation: Gethsemani Talks* (Singapore: Medio Media, 2007; updates published 2011).

Main, John. *Letters from the Heart: Christian Monasticism and the Renewal of Community* (New York, NY: The Crossroad Publishing Company, 1982).

Main, John. *Moment of Christ* (London: Darton, Longman & Todd, 1984).

Main, John. *The Present Christ* (London: Darton, Longman & Todd, 1985).

Merton, Thomas. *The Wisdom of the Desert* (New York, NY: New Directions, 1970).

Meyer, Marvin. *The Nag Hammadi Scriptures: The Revised and Updated Translation of Sacred Gnostic Texts* (New York, NY: HarperOne, 2007).

Nouwen, Henri J.M. *Eternal Seasons: A Spiritual Journey through the Church's Year* (ed. Michael Ford; Notre Dame, IN: Ave Maria Press, 2007).

Pagels, Elaine. *The Gnostic Gospels* (New York, NY: Vintage Books, 1989).

'The Discourse on the Eighth and Ninth' (Nag Hammadi Codex VI, 6), (trans. Marvin Meyer and Willis Barnstone) *Gnostic Society Library*, http://www.gnosis.org/naghamm/discourse-meyer.html (accessed 2 Mar. 2023).

Ward, Tess. *Alternative Pastoral Prayers: Liturgies and Blessings for Health and Healing, Beginnings and Endings* (Norwich: Canterbury Press, 2012).

Wimber, John and Kevin Springer. *Power Healing* (London: Hodder & Stoughton, 1986).

Wright, N.T. *Paul: A Biography* (San Francisco, CA: Harper-One, 2018).

Contact the Author

Find out more about Kate's books, blog *Faith, Life and Cancer*, TV show, online course and events, or contact her if you are interested in inviting Kate to speak at your church or group, via:

Website: www.katenicholas.co.uk
Facebook: KateNicholas7363
Instagram: @Katenicholai
Twitter: @KateNicholas

If you are now interested in taking your story-telling a stage further and writing a book about your faith journey, you may also be interested in Kate's online course 'Write Your Soul Story: How to write your Christian autobiography or memoir'.

Write Your Soul Story
How to write your Christian autobiography or memoir

Ever thought about writing a book about your faith journey?
Not sure where to start?

Check out the online course at: www.katenicholas.co.uk/mysoulsstory

Notes

2. Waiting

[1] Henri J.M. Nouwen, *Eternal Seasons: A Spiritual Journey through the Church's Year* (ed. Michael Ford; Notre Dame, IN: Ave Maria Press, 2007), p. 38.

3. Numinous

[1] See Robert Browning (1812–89), 'Pippa's Song' (1841), *EnglishVerse.com* © 2021 https://englishverse.com/poems/pippas_song (accessed 24 Feb. 2023).

5. Rapha

[1] John Wimber and Kevin Springer, *Power Healing* (London: Hodder & Stoughton, 1986), p. 60.

[2] Alex Strangwayes-Booth, 'Three in Five British Adults Say Miracles Are Possible', *BBC News*, 30 Sept. 2018 https://www.bbc.co.uk/news/uk-45679730 (accessed 14 Feb. 2023).

[3] Charles Capps, *God's Creative Power® for Healing* (Broken Arrow, OK: Charles Capps Publishing, 1991), p. 14.

[4] *Encounter Prayer: A space to meet with the living God for relationship, healing, transformation* https://www.encounterprayer.net/.

6. Decisions

[1] From the *Carmina Gadelica* (the song of the Gauls or Celts).

7. Carcinos

[1] Jaime R. Herndon, 'The History of Cancer: Discovery and Treatment', *Very Well Health*, 11 Dec. 2022 https://www.very wellhealth.com/the-history-of-cancer-514101 (accessed 14 Feb. 2023).

10. Setting Sail

[1] Morning and Evening Prayer, *The Church of England: A presence in every community* https://www.churchofengland.org/prayer-and-worship/worship-texts-and-resources/common-worship/daily-prayer/morning-and-evening.

14. Silence

[1] *Songs from Taizé* copyright @ Ateliers et Presses de Taizé, 71250, Taizé, France.
[2] *Songs from Taizé*.

16. Holy Ground

[1] While increasingly there is acknowledgment among medics that prayer can help healing, many scientists would argue that you can't subject prayer to proper scientific analysis because it

is impossible to control for all the confounding variables – extra factors not accounted for – such as the fervency, worthiness and morality of those praying, as well as others outside the control group who might also be praying for the patient. Some Christians also find the idea of testing God's apparent ability and willingness to heal as abhorrent, and there's no doubt that the relationship between prayer and healing is a complex one.

2 Larry Dossey MD, *Healing Words: The Power of Prayer and the Practice of Medicine* (San Francisco, CA: HarperCollins Publishers, 1993), p. 97.
3 Dossey, *Healing Words*, p. 24.
4 'Prayer of Abandon', *Spiritual Family Charles de Foucauld* © 2023 Association Famille Spirituelle Charles de Foucauld https://www.charlesdefoucauld.org/en/priere.php (accessed 24 Feb. 2023).
5 Dossey, *Healing Words*, p. 24.
6 Bede Griffiths, *The Marriage of East and West* (Tucson, AZ: Medio Media, 1976), pp. 3–4.
7 Griffiths, *Marriage of East and West*, p. 199.
8 Daniel Nicholas, *Sort of Haiku*, 1991 (unpublished poems).
9 Griffiths, *Marriage of East and West*, p. 132.
10 Griffiths, *Marriage of East and West*, p. 132.

17. Ancient Paths

1 Marvin Meyer, ed., *The Nag Hammadi Scriptures: The Revised and Updated Translation of Sacred Gnostic Texts* (New York, NY: HarperOne, 2007), p. 139.
2 *The Discourse on the Eighth and Ninth* (Nag Hammadi Codex VI, 6), trans. Marvin Meyer and Willis Barnstone, Gnostic Society Library, *Gnosis Archive* http://www.gnosis.org/naghamm/discourse-meyer.html (accessed 24 Feb. 2023). Permission given by Willis Barnstone, Distinguished Professor Emeritus of Comparative Literature at Indiana University, Bloomington, IN. Author of *The Secret Reader: 501 Sonnets* and *The Gnostic Bible* (with Marvin Meyer).

18. Kingdom Glimpses

1   See Dylan Thomas, 'Do not go gentle into that good night', in *Dylan Thomas Omnibus: Under Milk Wood, Poems, Stories and Broadcasts* (London: Weidenfeld & Nicolson, 2014; first published 1995), p. 128.

2   Prayer 'Go on your journey from this world' by Tess Ward from *Alternative Pastoral Prayers: Liturgies and Blessings for Health and Healing, Beginnings and Endings* is © Tess Ward 2012 (Norwich: Canterbury Press, 2012), p. 289.

20. Solitude

1   Thomas Merton, *The Wisdom of the Desert* (New York, NY: New Directions, 1970), p. 6 [Copyright 1960 by The Abbey of Gethsemani Inc].

22. Exploration

1   N.T. Wright, *Paul: A Biography* (San Francisco, CA: HarperOne, 2018), p. 52. Reproduced with permission of the Licensor through PLSclear.

2   *The Cloud of Unknowing and Other Works* (trans. A.C. Spearing; London: Penguin Classics, 2001), p. x.

3   *The Bede Griffiths Sangha Newsletter*, p. 3.

4   Richard H.H. Johnston, Christian Mindfulness Course, Session 4.

5   Richard H.H. Johnston, *Introducing Christian Mindfulness* (self-published, 2015), p. 18.

23. Shoreline

1   *Common Worship: Services and Prayers for the Church of England*, Holy Communion, Order One (Prayer A), Church House Publishing © The Archbishops Council, 2000, p. 19.

2   *Common Worship: Services and Prayers for the Church of England*, Holy Communion, Order One (Prayer A), Church House Publishing © The Archbishops Council, 2000, p. 14.

3   From Laurence Freeman, 'Introduction', *John Main: Essential Writings. Selected with an introduction by Laurence Freeman* (Maryknoll, NY: Orbis Books, 2002), p. 25. Freeman is quoting from John Cassian's Tenth Conference.

4   *Cloud of Unknowing*, p. 62.

5   *Cloud of Unknowing*, p. 61.

6   *Cloud of Unknowing*, p. 29.

7   Freeman, *John Main: Essential Writings*, p. 19.

8   Freeman, *John Main: Essential Writings*, p. 27.

9   John Main, *Christian Meditation: Gethsemani Talks* (Singapore: Medio Media, 2007; updates published 2011), p. 45.

10 John Main, *Moment of Christ* (London: Darton, Longman & Todd, 1984), pp. 37–8.

11 Main, *Moment of Christ*, pp. 37–8.

12 Main, *Moment of Christ*, pp. 17–18.

13 Main, *Moment of Christ*, pp. xi–xii.

14 John Main, *The Present Christ* (London: Darton, Longman & Todd, 1985), p. 117.

15 John Main, *Letters from the Heart: Christian Monasticism and the Renewal of Community* (New York, NY: The Crossroad Publishing Company, 1982), pp. 95–6.

16 *Cloud of Unknowing*, pp. 51–2.

24. Black Dog

[1] Ken Curtis, *Reflections on the Beatitudes for People with Cancer: A Personal Journey Presented by Ken Curtis @* Vision Video (Worcester, PA: Vision Video, 2013).

26. Anticipation

[1] Jonathan Jackson, *The Mystery of Art: Becoming an Artist in the Image of God* (Chesterton, IN: Ancient Faith Publishing, 2014), pp. 30–31.

28. Aftermath

[1] Nicky Gumbel, 'Glorified in Defeat', Day 281, *The Bible in One Year* https://bibleinoneyear.org/en/ © Copyright Alpha International 2022.

Epilogue

[1] Nouwen, *Eternal Seasons*, p. 38.

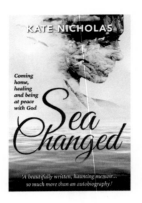

Sea Changed

Coming home, healing and being at peace with God

Kate Nicholas

Sea Changed is the vibrant account of an unconventional search for faith, truth and healing which reveals how God can be found in the most unexpected of places – even a cancer diagnosis.

Growing up with a strong sense of spirituality, Kate searched long and hard throughout the world to make sense of that spiritual longing. After catching glimpses of the divine in many cultures along the way, Kate finally found God and her life was transformed for ever.

Sea Changed tells the story of Kate's first battle with advanced breast cancer and her miraculous healing, along with other struggles such as the loss of both her parents, the loss of a baby, and debilitating ME.

This book encourages readers to recognise the unseen hand that shifts our perspective, alters our trajectory and lifts us up even in our darkest moments.

978-1-78078-162-4

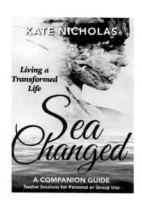

Sea Changed: A Companion Guide

Living a transformed life

Kate Nicholas

Transformation is foundational to our faith as followers of Christ. But what does it mean: living a transformed life?

Kate Nicholas helps us to understand how God is always actively transforming our lives; through his word, the promptings of the Holy Spirit and through the circumstances of our lives, and shows us what the fruits of this transformation look like.

Using a mix of biblical teaching, personal testimony and questions for reflection, Kate shows us how we can group to be more like him.

This twelve-session practical guide encourages us all to live a life transformed by God.

978-1-78078-996-5

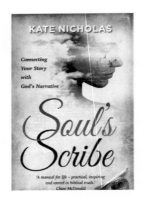

Soul's Scribe

Connecting your story with God's narrative

Kate Nicholas

Each of us has a soul story to tell – the unique story of how we experience God throughout our lives. This book is a guide to understanding and sharing your soul story.

Kate Nicholas expertly takes you on a journey through the various stages of your life, helping you to see your soul's story as an adventure full of meaning and purpose, connecting your tale with the great sweeping arc of God's eternal narrative.

As you identify the main themes of your life that connect past and present, you will be able to understand your life as a coherent whole. And at the end of this reflective and practical process, you will have the tools to step out and tell your own story with confidence.

Point others to Jesus as you are empowered to share the good things God has done for you.

978-1-78893-021-5

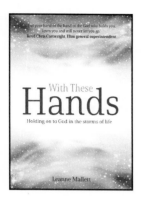

With These Hands

*Holding on to God
in the storms of life*

Leanne Mallett

Leanne's battle with breast cancer forced her to face some of her greatest fears and tested her faith in a way she had never experienced before. Treatment changed her appearance and stripped her of her identity as a woman, and her life was changed.

With deep honesty, Leanne shares how she dealt with this new reality and reveals the lessons she learned about God's incredible faithfulness and the strength that he gives us when we need it most.

978-1-78893-274-5

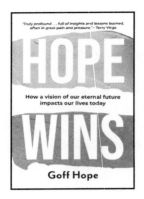

Hope Wins

How a vision of our eternal future
impacts our lives today

Goff Hope

Hope is fundamental for human wellbeing but it is in short supply in our world. We can quickly be robbed of hope by illness, personal tragedy or by the sheer oppressive nature of news headlines.

Drawing on his own personal experiences, including the tragedy of losing his daughter and his own battle with cancer, Goff shares how holding on to the Christian hope of an eternal future transformed the darkest moments of his life.

Interweaving personal testimony of the goodness of God with biblical teaching on heaven, Goff encourages us to see that when tough times come, and we are tempted to doubt or ask the big questions, such as Why, Lord?, we can have hope if we keep our eyes on Jesus and have a heavenly perspective on life.

978-1-78893-276-9

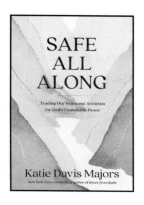

Safe All Along

Trading our fears and anxieties for God's unshakable peace

Katie Davis Majors

As a missionary, wife, and mum of fifteen, Katie Davis Majors knows how hard it can be to receive God's peace instead of giving in to fear and worry. Family emergencies, unexpected life-shifting events, and the busy rhythms of family life have at times left her reeling.

In *Safe All Along*, Katie offers reflections and stories from around the world and from her own kitchen table about her personal journey toward living from a place of surrendered trust. Every chapter leads us deep into Scripture as we learn what it looks like to break free from anxiety and take hold of peace.

Our God has promised us a peace that transcends all understanding. And we can accept his promise, trusting that in him we are safe all along.

978-1-78893-316-2

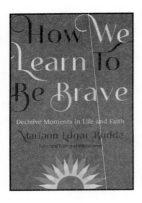

How We Learn to Be Brave

Decisive moments in life and faith

Mariann Edgar Budde

The decisive moments in life are those pivot points when we're called on to push past our fears and act with strength. Being brave is not a singular occurrence; it's a journey that we can choose to undertake every day.

Drawing on examples ranging from Harry Potter to the Gospel According to Luke, Budde seamlessly weaves together personal experiences with stories from Scripture, history, and pop culture to underscore both the universality of these decisive moments and the particular call each one of us must heed when they arrive.

How We Learn to Be Brave will provide much-needed fortitude and insight to anyone searching for answers in uncertain times.

978-1-78893-280-6

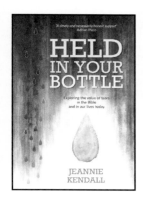

Held in Your Bottle

*Exploring the value of tears in the
Bible and in our lives today*

Jeannie Kendall

Whether we are crying tears of regret, loss, gratitude or anger the
Bible says that God holds them all in his bottle. We can draw comfort
from the fact that no tear goes unseen by him.

Each of these emotions is explored by a modern day story mirroring a
retelling of a relevant Bible character's experience. Insightful reflections then help us understand the issues raised.

Held in Your Bottle will enable you to look at the Bible in a fresh way
and help you accept and understand your emotional life.

978-1-78893-171-7

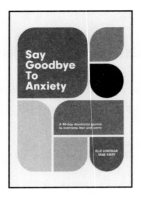

Say Goodbye to Anxiety

A 40-day devotional journal to overcome fear and worry

Elle Limebear and Jane Kirby

Anxiety has been calling the shots for too long. Enough is enough, it's time to say goodbye.

Elle and Jane get it. Having both suffered with anxiety, they understand how it can impact our daily lives. They also know the difference Jesus can make.

As they honestly share their story, Elle and Jane support and cheer us on as they offer God-given practical tools and strategies to overcome anxiety.

Be encouraged, through these 40 devotional thoughts and journaling reflections, to take daily steps with God's help to move past anxiety and live life to the full.

978-1-78893-312-4